Slim, Sane, and Sexy

Slim, Sane, and Sexy

Pocket Guide to
Natural, Bioidentical Hormone Balancing

by
JAY H. MEAD, MD
ERIN T. LOMMEN, ND

Calaroga Publishing
Oregon City, Oregon

Calaroga Publishing
619 Madison St #110
Oregon City, Oregon 97045
971-645-4068

Printed in the United States of America.
The cover is printed on 12 point Carolina/Productolith coated one side cover stock and contains 10% post consumer recycled content. The text is printed on 60# Natural Exact Opaque Recycled, Vellum paper containing 30% post consumer recycled content. The inks used are soy based.

ISBN: 978-0-9815793-0-6
Library of Congress Control Number: 2008923081

Editing: Kathryn A. Williams, MA, WordTurners.com
Interior Design & Typesetting: Jennifer Omner, ALLPublications.com

Disclaimer
Calaroga Publishing has created this book to provide information on the subject matters covered. Every effort has been made to make this book complete and accurate with the purpose of educating. It should be understood that the publisher and authors are not liable for the misconceptions or misuse of provided information. Neither Calaroga Publishing nor the authors are liable or responsible to any person or entity for direct or indirect loss, damage, or injury caused or allegedly caused by information contained in this book. The information presented herein is in no way intended as a substitute for medical counsel.

To Order
Visit www.slimsaneandsexy.com to order copies of the book online.

We dedicate this book to John R. Lee, MD, friend, colleague, and leader, whose pioneering research with natural hormones opened the door for the rest of us.

Contents

Acknowledgements

We are deeply indebted to Ann L. Hovland whose immense talent, wisdom, and clarity transformed our ideas into manuscript pages. We also gratefully acknowledge our gifted editor and writing consultant, Kate Williams of Wordturners, whose patience, diligence, and discipline made this book finally happen.

We owe a debt of gratitude to our patients, who by placing in us a sacred trust have fostered our understanding and expertise in bioidentical hormone therapies.

We would like to thank Jennifer Omner for the intelligent layout and design, as well as Nicole Weber for the sharp and intuitive graphics and illustrations. Thank you also to Cindy Barnhouse for the inspired artistry on cover design.

Finally, we both want to thank our families, as they are the foundation from which we move, making it all worthwhile. And Helena B. Lommen, thank you for your pioneering spirit and steadfast belief in treating the body naturally—it lives on. Thank you also to our mothers, Cleora Ann Mead and Donna Riveland Lommen, who imprinted in us the will to seek what is good and right in the world and the desire to further its understanding.

Preface

When we first met over a cup of coffee years ago, it was to find common ground and explore the idea of working together as clinicians—a medical doctor and a naturopathic physician. Jay, the MD, was in the middle of a professional transformation, seeking an-

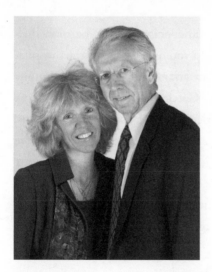

swers beyond the bounds of his conventional medical training. Erin, the ND, was looking for a clinical setting that offered her patients a full spectrum of options, including blending in conventional treatments. What we couldn't have known then was how far serendipity would take us. Here we are, nearly a decade later, partners in practice and life. Our marriage is, of course, a personal relationship, but it is also a metaphor for an exciting, holistic movement in health and healing. A blending of common sense, naturally-based therapies, and the diagnostic tools of modern medicine. This is not only a richly rewarding way to practice medicine, but more importantly, patients thrive.

Patient-centered medicine is our passion and our life's work. It is the motivating force behind this book.

In 20 years of practice, we have treated thousands of women between the ages of 35 and 65 who have been at wit's end with the ups and downs of hormonal fluctuations, and have found little, if any, relief from conventional approaches. There is hope and help for your symptoms and health beyond menopause, and our methods prove to be much safer than the commonly prescribed hormone replacement therapy (HRT).

Bioidentical hormone replacement therapy (BHRT) is revolutionizing women's comfort and health levels as they age. When used with a nutritious diet and regular exercise, bioidentical hormones can help relieve a long list of debilitating symptoms and restore a sense of well-being.

Slim, Sane, and Sexy is a clear and concise guide to hormone balancing. We have organized it to help you quickly access the information you need. If, for example, you are anxious to do something immediately, you can turn to Chapter 5 "Getting off the Edge: Correcting the Problem," which describes particular imbalances, their symptoms, and action steps. If you like to get a sense of the overall picture before taking action, starting at the beginning and reading the entire book will provide you the information needed to confidently move forward. However you use the book, it is our sincere hope that it provides you with powerful tools for taking charge of your health and your life!

Jay's Story

At 51, I still marvel at my impulse years ago to abandon a well-paying desk job with the American Red Cross for the uncertainties of establishing a clinical practice. After earning a degree from a prestigious medical school and successfully practicing pathology for 20 years, a nagging voice beckoned me to look deeper, to question my purpose. Although professionally successful, I had not yet fulfilled my potential as a healer—comforting those who are ill while helping alleviate their suffering.

For most of my career, I had ignored the faint voice. But that changed when I came face to face with my own mortality, when I learned I had a serious heart condition. Awakening to the preciousness of life and seeking healing myself was the motivation I needed to explore the healer within me. However, I didn't know where to begin. How after working in a lab and at a desk for so many years would I enter the world of clinical medicine?

The Chinese proverb "when the student is ready, the teacher appears" could not have been more true for me. Roy L. Swank, MD, famous for his multiple sclerosis diet and book on the subject, *The Multiple Sclerosis Diet Book*, invited me to join his practice. I decided to trust the voice and took the leap. Over the ensuing year, I saw several hundred patients with multiple sclerosis and learned a tremendous amount about how nutritional habits and the environment can impact health and healing. By following the Swank diet, which included reducing their intake of animal fat, patients substantially lowered their risk of recurrence of this devastating disease. Using a low saturated fat diet instead of pharmaceuticals to approach a chronic illness was a radical idea for me—certainly not in the scope of the mainstream medicine I had been taught in medical school. This experience opened my eyes and whetted my appetite for exploring other environmental causes of poor health.

It was also while working with Dr. Swank that I first encountered naturopathic medicine. A naturopathic medical student who was observing Dr. Swank's practice talked about using nutrition and natural remedies to treat chronic disease. As my contacts and interests in natural medicine grew, I ended up teaching pathology at the nearby naturopathic medical college, further immersing me in holistic natural medicine. I soon discovered that natural remedies were more effective and far less toxic than any treatments I had studied in conventional medical school. At the same time, I was also discovering organizations of medical doctors who practiced complementary medicine.

All of these influences eventually led me to open my own clinic, the Center for Integrative Medicine. I was finally home. Within a few weeks of launching my practice, I met Erin Lommen, ND, who had been practicing naturopathic medicine for 15 years. She graciously joined the clinic and helped fill in the gaps in my natural medicine knowledge, allowing us to offer patients a truly integrative medical approach.

One of the areas that both Erin and I were keenly interested in was hormone balancing. John R. Lee, MD, prolific author and pioneer of bioidentical hormone therapy, taught us both about the benefits of natural progesterone and how important it is to tailor hormone preparations to individual patient needs. As a result we have helped hundreds if not thousands of patients using Dr. Lee's teachings on bioidentical hormone replacement.

Since Dr. Lee's death in 2003, numerous spokespersons for bioidentical hormones have stepped up. But we have been disturbed by the amount of misinformation and even dangerous advice that has ensued. Not all of the claimed experts have the facts right. On the basis of our training and clinical experience, we have written this book to provide accurate, current information on bioidentical hormones. We are committed to Dr. Lee's approach and have the support of Pat Lee, his wife of 44 years and our dear friend, to continue and extend his work.

It is my hope that medical school curricula and other disenchanted MDs will break out of the conventional medical model and embrace complementary, natural medical principles and practices. I continue to listen to my inner voice in ever-deeper ways, as it never completely rests. My mission now is to share what I know and practice in harmony with the Hippocratic oath tenet: above all, do no harm.

Erin's Story

As a young girl, I would watch, fascinated, as my grandmother brushed her long silver, silken hair, take the waist-length strands, braid them, and then wrap it all into a bun. She never had her haircut, ever. As I grew, I learned there were many more ways she resisted convention, medicine being one of them. Raised by the first compounding pharmacist in the Dakota Territory, she learned about natural therapies and the body's inherent healing wisdom. She took that wisdom with her as a nurse during World War I.

Using natural therapies for healing, my grandmother raised four children without the aid of conventional medicine, leaving a legacy of trust in the power of nature to heal. Admiring her so deeply, I took this trust to heart and in that my desire to work with the body to support its healing grew. To this day, I keep one of her medical books (originally her father's) on my desk in our office: *Colon Hygiene* by John Harvey Kellogg—a natural healer whom I learned about during my naturopathic medical training.

I was also greatly impacted by an event with my maternal grandfather who had been hospitalized for respiratory complaints while my parents were away traveling. I was 18 years old at the time and uncertain about my direction, but was attending college with a medical career in mind.

I visited my grandfather in the hospital. He was lying on top of the bed fully dressed with shoes on uttering swear words under his breath.

I said, "Bestefar (Norwegian for grandfather) are you all right?" While relieved to see me, he made clear his anger about the situation and the staff he was forced to depend upon. Infuriated, he explained how abrupt the move had been from his retirement home to the hospital, as well as the caregiver's lack of respect. He said he was freezing and that his feet were so cold they were blue. He had refused to put on the hospital gown.

I confronted the nurses with this information, and they rolled their eyes while describing to me how this confused old man was behaving impossibly. When I spoke to his doctor, I learned that my grandfather was on a new medication for dementia. It turned out that the dementia medication had been causing the confusion and incoherence, and once it was removed he resumed his life at the nursing home free from these symptoms for many more years.

This experience ignited a desire to be involved in a type of medical care that recognizes each individual as unique and substantial. It encouraged me to seek a form of healing that would not interfere with the body but instead would work with it to initiate and promote healing.

I continued down an academic path to become a conventional medical doctor, completing a pre-med degree in my undergraduate studies. However, in considering conventional medical school, I couldn't help questioning the conflicts I felt between my experiences and the predominant approach used in conventional medicine—symptom-based and specialist-driven. How could I practice a medicine that did not value the whole body or whole person when diagnosing or treating?

Shortly before completing my bachelor's degree, I participated in a rotation with a respiratory therapist. My experience that evening made it clear I could not pursue this form of medicine. We had addressed numerous patients, and it was not an unusual shift. In the conventional medical language of symptom-focused treatment, we attended a pneumothorax and an MI, among others. As you might imagine, nowhere was I able to find the central core of these patients' care, where the whole person was evaluated and treated. The concern was not about how these people ended up with lung disease and heart disease, or whether or not they could reverse it or heal any of it. I couldn't help wondering if there were other seemingly unrelated things happening in their bodies that were contributing. Filled with questions and doubts, I abandoned my dream of attending a conventional medical school.

Three years later, while waiting tables in a restaurant, I was casting about for a new career direction when I was introduced to a different approach to medicine—naturopathic medicine. A fellow waiter announced one evening that he was going to become a doctor the next day. I began asking questions and learned from him that he would be graduating with a Doctorate of Naturopathic Medicine degree (ND) from the National College of Naturopathic Medicine (currently National College of Natural Medicine) in Portland, Oregon. As fate would have it, I actually had been living next door to that college. At the time, it was one of only two naturopathic medical schools in the country. (There are now five in the United States and two in Canada.)

It took three years and some extensive planning, researching, and questioning before I enrolled. I had found a form of medical practice that incorporated the healing wisdom of nature and honored the Hippocratic tenet: do no harm. In pursuing naturopathic medicine, my conflicts and doubts about practicing medicine were resolved. After graduating in 1989, I went into private practice.

My advance into using bioidentical hormones came with the advent of saliva testing as a diagnostic tool. Evaluating individual's saliva constituents provided greater clinical information about hormone imbalances than blood tests. I had been practicing a couple of years when I began testing adrenal function using saliva tests, enhancing my ability to help individuals suffering from a myriad of diseases and dysfunctions. In less than 10 years, individual female and male hormone balancing using bioidentical hormones followed naturally as saliva testing progressed and developed accuracy in profiling hormone levels.

Because of my focus on women's health and the intricate role hormones play, incorporating bioidentical hormone replacement therapy has been a great asset to my practice. Personally experiencing the benefits of natural hormones as I age, I feel fundamentally committed to offering safe alternatives to conventional HRT. As well, having a mother diagnosed with breast cancer brought home the importance of finding and using safe hormone replacement therapies for my patients and myself.

During this time I met Jay at the Natural College of Naturopathic Medicine, where we were both teaching as associate professors. Together we created a successful integrative clinic, The Center for Integrative Medicine, and have since helped hundreds of female patients get balanced with natural bioidentical hormone therapies. Because of our desire to further advance bioidentical therapies and as a natural evolution of our friendship with the late John R. Lee, MD, we also started a medical laboratory, Labrix Clinical Services, Inc., specifically aimed at the accurate and precise evaluation of hormone levels using saliva testing.

After nearly 20 years as a practitioner of naturopathic medicine, I continue to be awed by the power of the naturopathic principles. I remain a humble lifelong student of their guiding wisdom.

Principles of Naturopathic Medicine

The Healing Power of Nature

Naturopathic medicine recognizes an inherent ability in the body, which is ordered and intelligent. Naturopathic physicians act to identify and remove obstacles to recovery and to facilitate and augment this healing ability.

Identify and Treat the Causes

The naturopathic physician seeks to identify and remove the underlying causes of illness, rather than to eliminate or merely suppress symptoms.

First Do No Harm

Naturopathic medicine follows three principles to avoid harming the patient:

- Utilize methods and medicinal substances that minimize the risk of harmful side effects.
- Avoid, when possible, the harmful suppression of symptoms.
- Acknowledge and respect the individual's healing process, using the least force necessary to diagnose and treat illness.

Doctor as Teacher

Naturopathic physicians educate the patient and encourage self-responsibility for health. They also acknowledge the therapeutic value inherent in the doctor-patient relationship.

Treat the Whole Person

Naturopathic physicians treat each individual by taking into account physical, mental, emotional, genetic, environmental, social, and other factors. Since total health also includes spiritual health, naturopathic physicians encourage individuals to pursue their personal spiritual path.

Prevention

Naturopathic physicians emphasize disease prevention, assessment of risk factors, and hereditary susceptibility to disease and making appropriate interventions to prevent illness. Naturopathic medicine strives to create a healthy world in which humanity may thrive.

Introduction
Is Hormone Havoc
Pushing You to the Edge?

Despite managing menstrual cycles and hormone fluctuations for decades, entering mid-life can often leave you overwhelmed by new, seemingly inexplicable, physical and emotional symptoms. Symptoms that make you wonder whether you are going to lose the last toe-hold on emotional balance, mental sharpness, physical youthfulness, and well-being. Dogged by self-doubt and anxiety, at mid-life you can feel abandoned and betrayed, searching for lost confidence and a familiar self.

Competent, accomplished women can find themselves wrestling with levels of insecurity not experienced since the rocky days of puberty. To make matters worse, their bodies can begin to betray them. Skin wrinkles and sags, hair grays and grows brittle, and sex can become uninteresting or routine.

Sound familiar? Do you as a mid-life woman just need to accept these changes? Is your former self destined to dry up and whither away after 40? Is this the beginning of the end? Of course not.

Armed with the right information, you can stay vital, sexy, and empowered through your mid-life transition on into your 70s, 80s, and beyond. The years from age 35 to 55 are, actually, a portal to a new phase of life, a birthing of the wise years to come. Rather than an end-point, it is a beginning, a reward for all of the hard lessons of your early years. What seems like a shear drop-off is rather an edge signaling you to spread your wings. With a little support and a trust that your wings will withstand the transient turbulence of shifting hormones, you can soar into the next phase of life. Balancing your hormones naturally and safely can smooth this transition, while enhancing your health in the second half of life. Getting your hormone levels accurately tested and having a trained physician prescribe bioidentical hormones specifically compounded to correct your particular imbalance can accomplish this goal.

Do You Relate?

- Trouble falling asleep or wake up in the night?
- Less able to handle stress?
- More difficulty making decisions?
- Increased criticism of self and others?
- Obsessive thinking and worrying?
- Uncharacteristic memory loss and foggy thinking?

A Word About The Change

Today women are likely to live more than half of their lives after menopause. Women born in 2005 in the United States have a life expectancy of 80 years; women live the longest in Japan, where their life expectancy is nearly 86 years. On average in industrialized nations women can expect to live into their upper seventies to lower eighties.[1]

This modern reality has created a dilemma: women are far outliving their historic biological timelines. Four hundred years ago, a woman could only expect to live, on average, to the age of 35. Even as recently as 1900, life expectancy was only 47 years old.[2] Perhaps this was due, in part, to high infant and childhood mortality. Nonetheless, women who made it to menopause had already outlived their life expectancy. No wonder "the change" was seen as a death sentence. Even though women's lives no longer end around menopause, archaic perceptions of that time are alive and well, so much so that women often deny it is happening.

While liberated women of our generation have sought to take charge of their bodies, they are, ironically, often in denial when it comes to this change. Regardless of women's personal or individual orientation to aging within social tradition, menopause marks a loss of women's currency of power—youthful beauty and the ability to bear children. Whether or not this is true for you personally, these attributes often form the core of women's identity, containing potent social and political ramifications. Middle-aged women coming into our office often report feeling like they have become invisible in the world. If she hasn't already, as menopause and its hormonal changes approach, a woman must grapple with establishing a new point of reference for her place in the world.

Remember, menopause is a natural process. Biologically, our youthfully beautiful bodies are geared to attract a mate and reproduce. Once that has been accomplished, our bodies become expendable and gradually begin to wind down their systems through the aging process.

The good news is we can improve the quality of our lives as that process unfolds. There are healthful, safe ways to leverage the physiology of aging, to reclaim the vitality levels formerly relinquished to the young. We can live longer, be attractive, and age gracefully into our 90s and beyond. Aging is, in fact, hastened by a number of hormone deficiencies. The first step in correcting these deficiencies and imbalances is to identify some symptoms.

Signs of Hormone Havoc

The ways women experience hormone imbalances are as varied as women themselves. Symptoms can be physical, mental, emotional, or more likely a combination of them all. These are some of the common signs:

- You feel like you are on an emotional roller coaster—feelings are fragile, raw, and unpredictable. One minute you may be extremely irritated by small details and the next, on the verge of tears. Anxiety and panic episodes may have ballooned out of control.

- You are tired all of the time and find you are gaining weight while eating the same diet.

- Self-doubt and brain fog have taken on new extremes—the occasional memory lapse is now an everyday occurrence.

- You find yourself repeatedly awake at 4:00 a.m.—sometimes in a cold or hot sweat.

- You're hanging by your fingernails, scared that friends, family, and co-workers suspect you're incompetent or even crazy.

How Are Your Hormones Doing?

For a preliminary look at whether hormone imbalances may be affecting your health and sense of well-being, take the following quick survey.

Yes	No	
☐	☐	Hot flashes/night sweats
☐	☐	Sleeplessness
☐	☐	Bleeding irregularities/menstrual changes
☐	☐	Unwanted hair growth
☐	☐	Scalp hair loss
☐	☐	Weight gain (especially around the middle)
☐	☐	Low sex drive/less orgasms
☐	☐	Thinning skin/increased wrinkling
☐	☐	Joint pain and stiffness
☐	☐	Breast lumps
☐	☐	Migraine headaches
☐	☐	Depression
☐	☐	Bone loss

Total ___ ___

If you checked "yes" for two or more symptoms, it is likely you have a hormone imbalance that bioidentical hormones can help correct. For more clues about which hormones are the likely offenders, you will find the more in-depth "Hormone Pretest" on page 83.

You Can Do Something About It

If you suspect hormone fluctuations are causing at least some of the havoc in your life, the question is what can you do about it. With the insights and guidance provided in this book, plenty.

Although you may be finding yourself teetering on the edge of no return, opening this book will break your fall and send you moving ahead on a new, exciting path. You are taking the first step across the abyss, opening up a world of possibilities for the adventure that is the rest of your life. *Slim, Sane, and Sexy* is your clear roadmap to safe, healthful hormonal balance and lifestyle enhancing practices.

What You Can Have at Any Age . . .

- Robust sensuality and an active sex life
- Svelte, appropriate-shaped body for your genetics and bone structure
- Serene, content disposition
- A good night's sleep
- Creative, playful outlook
- Strong, wise attitude
- Active, athletic lifestyle
- Vitality for any activity
- Curiosity

Read On and You Will

- ▶ discover whether you have a hormonal imbalance;
- ▶ identify your imbalance;
- ▶ find out how bioidentical hormones can help;
- ▶ optimize hormone levels without attempting to recreate the menstrual cycle, which poses risks for breast, endometrial, and ovarian cancers;

- ▶ learn the right way to use bioidentical hormones;
- ▶ discover how lifestyle choices can support hormone balance;
- ▶ take action to relieve your particular symptoms;
- ▶ gain a better understanding of the aging process;
- ▶ find using bioidentical hormones during perimenopause a catalyst for turning back the clock;
- ▶ take charge of your life and well-being again;
- ▶ realize you can be as slim, sane, and sexy as you want to be.

◄ 1 ►
Why Bioidentical Hormones?

Chances are you have heard something about bioidentical hormones over the past few years. There has been a steady stream of books and articles about this alternative to conventional hormone replacement therapy (HRT) since Dr. John Lee published his first book on the subject in 1993, *Natural Progesterone: The Multiple Roles of a Remarkable Hormone*. Recently there has been a lot of press questioning the safety of conventional HRT and its link to breast cancer and heart problems. Concern over turf and financial losses have seemingly led the pharmaceutical industry, particularly Wyeth Pharmaceuticals, to strategically launch a public relations campaign against the safety and efficacy of bioidentical hormone therapy.[3,4,5] What is all the fuss about? Who is right? How are bioidentical hormones different from conventional hormone replacement therapy? And what, if anything, makes bioidentical hormones the better choice?

Broken Promises

Feminine Forever was the promise and title of Dr. Robert Wilson's book, published in 1966. In it he expresses his "sympathy" for women who are "condemned to witness the death of their own womanhood." He urges women to take the new wonder drug, Premarin to "remain

fully feminine—physically and emotionally—for as long as they live."
Dr. Wilson is given credit for defining menopause as "an estrogen-
deficiency disease," which became, and remains, the mantra in medical school training.[6] We now know this understanding is simplistic,
and even dangerous. The book followed Dr. Wilson's 1964 article on
menopause in Newsweek magazine.[7] The 170% growth of Premarin
sales between 1963 and 1966 is attributed to his writings and speaking tours extolling the virtues of Premarin. In 2002, Ronald Wilson,
Robert Wilson's son, reported that Wyeth Pharmaceuticals, the mak-
ers of Premarin, had financially supported his father's research foundation, book, and speaking tours. This conflict of interest was never men-
tioned in Dr. Wilson's writings. One might assume that corporations
are tasked with paying attention to the bottom line and stockholder's
dividends, while a government body such as the U.S. Food and Drug
Administration (FDA) protects the public from a harmful drug and
misinformation. Not true.

You will be disappointed if you assume that the Food and Drug
Administration is looking after our best interests. They can be as con-
flicted as their corporate bedfellows, evidenced by results found in
the 2002 Women's Health Initiative (WHI) study, and the Million
Women Study done in the United Kingdom between 1996 and 2001.
Between the two studies, they have confirmed that synthetic or conventional hormone replacement therapy increases a woman's risk for
breast, ovarian, and endometrial cancer, as well as heart disease.[8,9]

In fact, the WHI study was stopped early because of mounting evidence that one of the drugs used, PremPro, was increasing the subjects'
risk of breast cancer, heart disease, stroke, and blood clots in the lungs.
PremPro is a combination of Premarin (pregnant mare's urine) and
Provera (synthetic progesterone called progestin), which had been ap-
proved by the FDA for decades prior to these studies. When the news

hit the public media in 2002, large numbers of women justifiably abandoned PremPro. And guess what happened to the rate of breast cancer? As reported by researchers from the M.D. Anderson Cancer Center at the University of Texas, breast cancer rates declined an astonishing 7 percent in 2003.[10] This means there were 14,000 fewer breast cancer cases than predicted. This decline is directly attributed to the drop in PremPro usage. An additional factor may be at play here, however. We know from clinical practice that many women switched to bioidentical hormones after the study was publicized, further contributing to a reduction in PremPro risk factors. (The number of women who switched to bioidentical hormone therapy was not addressed in this study).

Not only has the FDA not protected women from the harmful effects of non-human hormones such as those in PremPro, corporate influence on the FDA decisions likely kept a much less expensive generic alternative from reaching the public. On May 5, 1997, the FDA acted against the public interest by blocking the application of a company proposing to produce a generic form of Premarin. This maneuver essentially gave American Home Products a monopoly on a billion-dollar market.[11]

The Conventional Myth:
Synthetic vs. Bioidentical Hormones

First let's clear up a question of semantics. We use the term "bioidentical" to describe human-identical hormones; these two terms are interchangeable. Even though bioidentical hormones replicate nature, calling them natural hormones is bit of a misnomer. The term "natural" generally refers to substances found in the plant world. There are similar forms found in plants, but none are human-identical. They do, however, provide the source for bioidentical hormones. These plant-based or phytohormones are chemically altered to precisely mirror the structure of human hormones. Bioidentical progesterone and estrogen, for example, can be created from chemically altered forms of the naturally occurring phytohormones found in the Mexican wild yam, soy, and other plants. In fact, all of the sex hormones and cortisol (adrenal gland energy hormone) are available in bioidentical forms.

How Do Bioidentical Hormones Compare with Synthetic Hormones?

Just because HRT is widely used doesn't mean it's safe or effective. The hormones used in conventional hormone replacement therapy are synthetic compounds developed and patented by pharmaceutical companies. For example, a synthetic component of PremPro is medroxy-progesterone or MP (MP falls within a group of synthetic molecules known as progestins or progestogens). This group mimics only some, not all, of the functions of human progesterone. Synthetically made hormones are not human identical.

One way to understand the limitations of a synthetic hormone is to contrast it to the human-identical hormone, progesterone. Progesterone acts like a master key that opens all of the doors to essential bodily functions controlled by this remarkable hormone, providing many benefits. On the other hand, a progestin is a key that opens only some doors to body functions, limiting its benefits. It may protect the uterus from the effects of too much estrogen, reducing the risk for cancer of the uterine lining (endometrium), but as shown in the Women's Health Initiative Study and the Million Women Study, it can be a risk factor in other potentially fatal diseases like breast and uterine cancer, and heart disease.

On the other hand, bioidentical progesterone not only protects the endometrium, it protects the breast from excess estrogen and performs other routine biologic functions such as maintaining bone density, protecting the cardiovascular system from hardening of the arteries (atherosclerosis), facilitating sleep, enhancing cognition, and having calming effects without any of the potentially deadly side effects of progestins.

One of the criticisms we hear about bioidentical hormone usage is that the long-term potential for harmful side effects has not been studied. That is true from the perspective of random controlled trials popularized by the pharmaceutical industry. It is not true if you consider what we know about the evolution of our species. Bioidentical hormones create us and sustain us. As these hormones decline or become imbalanced or both, we experience disease and effects of aging. If these hormones were harmful, the human species simply would not exist.

Consider also the development of a human embryo. The placenta that each of us was attached to through the umbilical cord produced estriol (a protective estrogen) and progesterone at levels that exceed adult levels by factors of ten to a hundred times. Yes, up to 100 times as much. As developing embryos, each of us was bathed in and swallowed these hormones for months. On what basis can one argue that these hormones taken in amounts that pale in comparison with what we were exposed to in utero could possibly be harmful to an adult human over a long term? This is what I heard a wise physician once call the sniff test. If common sense overwhelmingly refutes the argument, it passes the sniff test. All bioidentical hormones pass the test with flying colors.

Medicines don't necessarily require sophisticated, expensive controlled trials to confirm they are effective. Dr. N. A. Kurtzman wrote,

> It is useful to reflect on what an RCT [random controlled trial] tells us. It differentiates between a treatment that doesn't work and one that barely works and between treatments that differ very slightly. If the treatment is a great

advance, its effect is so obvious that an RCT is not necessary. . . . It is virtually axiomatic that the effectiveness of a
treatment is inversely proportional to the number of controlled studies that surround it.[12]

Bioidentical hormones perform in the same way our human hormones do, because they are no different in structure.

Unfortunately, most physicians are not aware of the distinction between progesterone and MP or, for that matter, the myriad of other
synthetically produced progestins that millions of women are exposed
to each day through treatment for birth control, PMS, or postmenopausal symptoms. Progesterone is distinct and not to be confused with
progestins. Aside from MP, several other progestins have also recently
been shown to have the same or higher incidence of side effects.[13]

Beyond the distinctions of origins and human compatibility between synthetic and bioidentical HRT, the associated methods of prescribing are vastly different. As stated previously, conventional medical
schools teach that menopause is a deficiency of estrogen—a false as-
sumption founded on 1960s writings by Dr. Robert Wilson's.[14] Continuing his misinformed theories into the 70s, Wilson wrote,

> At birth the ovaries contain an average of 4 million germ
> cells. At age 18 only 155,000 remain. At age 40 only about
> 8,300 are left and by age 50 there are only a few, perhaps not
> a single one, remaining—*no ova, no follicles, no theca cells,*
> *no estrogen*; truly a galloping catastrophe . . . The estrogenic
> treatment of older women will inhibit osteoporosis and
> thus help to prevent fractures . . . Breasts and genital organs
> will not shrivel. Such women will be much more pleasant
> to live with and will not become dull and unattractive.[15]

Guided by these assumptions, physicians prescribing conventional
HRT typically write standard prescriptions without first knowing
a woman's baseline hormone levels. Conventional medical training

teaches that all postmenopausal women need estrogen, and need it in the same dosages.

Dr. John Lee dispels this myth in all of his writings including his book, *What Your Doctor May Not Tell You About Menopause.*[16] After testing thousands of perimenopausal and menopausal women's hormone levels, this generalization is simply not true. Our experience is that every woman's hormone picture is different and most women have sufficient levels of estrogen, while, comparatively, their progesterone levels are waning. Therefore, we strongly recommend that you have your hormone levels tested before beginning any hormone therapy program.

The Healthier More Effective Choice

Bioidentical hormones are effective. By mimicking your body's own hormone molecules in structure and action, they provide a natural boost to nudge your own hormones back into balance. Identically matching our body's natural hormones, bioidentical hormones replicate, at the cellular level, the action of hormones naturally produced by the ovaries and adrenal glands.

The body's sex hormones—estrogen, testosterone, and progesterone—are in a continuous, interactive relationship with one another, "the dance of the steroids," to quote Dr. Lee. Since all hormone levels drop as we age, disrupting this hormone dance; determining your own hormone imbalance or deficiency and judiciously supplementing with bioidentical hormones will allow you to restore balance, turning back the clock on your aging process and its related symptoms.

The Safer Option

As we have said, bioidentical hormones are safer than conventional HRT because they are a precise replicate of the chemical structure of the hormones produced by your ovaries, adrenal, pituitary, and thyroid glands. Studies conducted in Europe suggest that bioidentical molecules are far safer than their synthetic counterparts because the body recognizes them as its own hormones.[17] Consequently bioidentical molecules take appropriate action, filling the appropriate site receptors, and efficiently breaking down into non-toxic metabolites.

Our cells have regions that act as receptor sites on their membranous surfaces. These receptors recognize hormones and capture them when they are available. Once within the receptor's grasp, the hormone enters the cell, eventually making its way into the master region, or nucleus, which maintains all of the genetic information and machinery to create the messengers that direct the cell function. The messengers initiate the production of proteins, the workhorses of each cell. The proteins produced are specific to the hormone that triggered their creation and cause the cell to alter its function accordingly. Like your own, when you had adequate levels, bioidentical hormone balancing leads to improved cell function, which enhances the overall performance of the body; for example, weight loss, increased vitality and energy, mood stabilization, improved muscle tone, better sugar metabolism, stronger bones, and improved sexual function.

By contrast, synthetic pharmaceuticals, such as conventional HRT drugs, must be molecularly altered, however slightly, changing the structure from that of the natural hormone in order for pharmaceutical companies to patent them and establish proprietary status and financial gain. Consequently, a patented hormone therapy can only provide a partial function of your native hormone, while at the same time putting you at risk for possible deadly side effects.

Do Bioidentical Hormones Have Any Side Effects?

Bioidentical hormones can have side effects when taken in excess of physiologic doses. If excess bioidentical estrogen is taken, for example, the imbalance produced could lead to increased risk of breast cancer, weight gain, mood changes, and tender breasts; likewise excess testosterone can cause scalp hair loss, acne, and facial hair. These side effects are the result of imbalance rather than incompatibility with human physiology, as in the side effects seen with synthetic hormones. When your own estrogen or testosterone is above normal levels for reasons we will discuss later, the same side effects will result. This is why you should always have your hormone levels tested before taking any hormone supplement—even bioidentical hormones.

Accurate and reliable testing will help establish the exact nature and extent of your hormone deficiencies, assuring that you take the correct physiologic doses within a safe, effective treatment regimen. Before you begin treatment, it is critical to both get tested and locate a health care provider to help tailor a treatment program that fits your hormone picture (*see* "Chapter 5, Getting Tested and Getting Support"). It is important to be guided and regularly monitored when using hormones. Remember, it is about creating the right balance for *you*, establishing your correct physiologic dosage.

A Custom Fit

Unlike conventional HRT, the most critical advantage of bioidentical hormones is ability to be tailored to your individual need. In the dynamic world of hormone balance, one size does not fit all. For example, if you are deficient in more than one hormone, a compounding pharmacist can formulate a single prescription for you that includes the unique mix of hormones you need in the right dosages. This is not the case with synthetic hormone replacement therapy, which is a one-size-fits-all approach. Every woman gets the same prescription, often estrogen alone with no progesterone to balance it.

What is a Compounding Pharmacist?

A compounding pharmacist is educated and licensed as any other pharmacist, but has extended training in creating or compounding custom medicines. Compounding pharmacists make medications from scratch using raw chemicals, powders, and devices. This includes preparing customized dosage forms and prescription medications that meet an individual patient or physician's needs. Before the industrial revolution 100 percent of physician prescriptions were formulated or compounded from raw ingredients by the local pharmacist. That percentage of compounded prescriptions dropped to 80% in 1920, 20% by 1940, and 1% in 1970.[18] For the most part pharmacists' roles changed throughout the twentieth century from an apothecary or chemist to a dispenser of manufactured dosage forms. Recently, however, there has been a resurgence of compounding pharmacists as patients and doctors are again realizing the benefits of individualized dosage forms and their place in treating patients' unique needs.

If Bioidentical Hormones Are So Great, Why Don't Most MDs Prescribe Them?

Bioidentical hormones cannot be patented, and, therefore, do not have the potential to generate high profits for drug companies. The pharmaceutical industry has shareholders who thrive on big profit margins—the kind of profits generated by patented drugs. A patent limits production to the patent-holding company and essentially creates a monopoly for that particular drug. Thus, there is tremendous incentive for drug companies to create drugs that can be patented—whether or not it is in the best interest of patients, as we pointed out earlier. Once a drug is created, companies must find or develop a market for it, which is why we are constantly bombarded with advertising for the latest and greatest drugs. You only have to turn on the TV to find a new pill that promises to make us happier, sexier, calmer, or more restful.

Patent law prohibits patenting naturally occurring elements, chemicals, or minerals. Drugs must include a new chemical entity (NCE), which is a novel molecule that does not exist in nature. Without a patent, bioidentical hormones are not a compelling product for drug companies. While not compelling to produce, pharmaceutical companies are acutely aware of needing to compete against products they cannot control through patents. In reaction to this burgeoning competition, the pharmaceutical industry appears to be making an effort to discredit bioidentical hormones and the pharmacists who prepare them.

On October 6, 2005, the pharmaceutical giant, Wyeth, filed a citizens petition with the FDA seeking to close pharmacies compounding bioidentical hormone replacement therapy (BHRT) drugs.[19] They claim that bioidentical hormones are not proven to be effective through randomized controlled research trials. As discussed above, when a remedy is clearly effective—and bioidentical hormones are effective—there is no need for controlled trials. More importantly, the primary drug used in conventional HRT, PremPro, is a huge profit maker for Wyeth. It has been on the market for decades and Wyeth has a vested interest in protecting market share. Women's and physician's response to the Women's Health Initiative Study and the Million Women Study outcomes have obviously imposed on business as usual in the pharmaceutical industry.

If the lack of controlled studies for bioidentical hormones still makes you uncomfortable, consider this insight: After years of practice and continuing education, it is apparent that well over two thirds of medical therapies have never been tested via controlled trials. Furthermore, the majority of drugs have unknown mechanisms of action according to the *Physicians' Desk Reference*. Controlled trials are a relatively recent convention to monitor the pharmaceutical industry. It is a precaution to protect the public, because most pharmaceuticals are not natural, or naturally derived, and have the potential for devastating or deadly side effects.

We have seen hundreds of patients find a profoundly enhanced quality of life through bioidentical hormone balancing. Your body identifies them as if they were their own. When monitored through definitive testing methods and prescribed in physiological doses, bioidentical hormones can be the answer to alleviating unwanted symptoms and accelerated aging.

Before exploring the types of imbalances and how to treat them, let's consider how your hormones became imbalanced and the contributing factors involved. As we get older our hormones predictably decrease, but there are factors that enhance this fall, prematurely initiate them, or create inappropriate levels in relation to our other sex hormones. These are factors we have some control over when making lifestyle and dietary choices.

◂ 2 ▸
How You Got Here
The Inside Story

While hormone imbalance has been around as long as women have had menstrual cycles, more and more women are experiencing symptoms earlier in life, and these symptoms are more debilitating than ever before. Why is this? There are likely many causes—our environment, food additives in the food chain, and the pace of twenty-first century life. All of these stress a woman's hormonal cycle. And the more stressors there are, the more likely you will experience severe hormonal swings. These swings are the cause of a myriad of seemingly unrelated symptoms, causing even more distress. If that is not enough to handle, the physiological weaknesses you bring with you into menopause may cause you even more dramatic symptoms.

Understanding the Hormone Dance

Each woman is born with a finite number of eggs (ova) in her ovaries. The body selects one or more eggs for possible fertilization during each menstrual cycle. While it is not known exactly *how* the body makes this selection, it *is* known that complex hormonal messengers initiate the cycle in the brain. These messengers are released into the bloodstream and find their way to the ovaries, where they direct the selection and eventual maturation and release of an egg (ovulation).

For most women, this process occurs in monthly cycles of approximately 28 days. The first part of the cycle is called the follicular phase because the developing egg is referred to as the follicle. The developing egg (follicle) is the primary source of estrogen and progesterone— it actually creates these hormones. When released, progesterone and estrogen become dance partners that serve clear, and in some ways opposite, functions throughout a woman's menstrual cycle. Estrogen is dominant during the first half of the cycle (days 1 to 15), giving tissues the message to grow or multiply to prepare the lining of the uterus for the egg. Once ovulation occurs (approximately day 15), estrogen levels drop and the developing egg ruptures through the surface of the ovary (ovulation).

Progesterone then takes center stage, blocking any further growth effects of estrogen on the endometrium or uterine lining. It also alters the endometrium so that a fertilized egg can implant and have the necessary nutrients to grow. Around day 25 of the menstrual cycle, the progesterone level falls back to baseline, or non-ovulatory levels causing the uterine lining to slough off resulting in menstruation.

This hormone synchronicity continues throughout a woman's menstrual life. However, the ratio of progesterone to estrogen steadily declines as a woman ages. Beginning at age 35, your balance begins to shift dramatically. This is because your developing eggs are not producing as much progesterone. It makes sense that the healthiest eggs are generally selected earlier in life, a kind of natural selection process. (Keep in mind it has only been within the last hundred years that a significantly higher percentage of women have even been alive to procreate into their fourth decade.) Estrogen production, on the other hand, usually does not drop in proportion to decreasing progesterone levels, which throws the balance off in favor of estrogen.

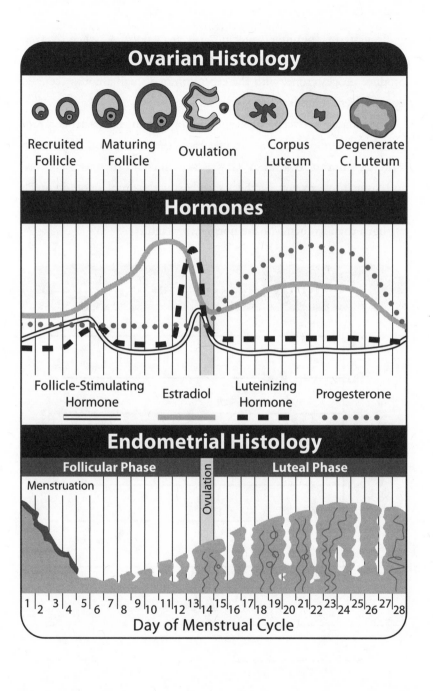

Progesterone plummets precipitously at menopause, when the ovaries essentially stop functioning altogether. Eventually, you no longer produce progesterone, with the exception of a small amount secreted by the adrenal glands.

The balance between estrogen and progesterone is further compromised by the fact that—as women age—the production of estrogen switches from the ovaries to fatty tissue, which, in turn, converts testosterone into estrogen, further exacerbating the problem of too much estrogen. Therefore, if you are overweight, you will produce even more estrogen than women who are normal in weight.

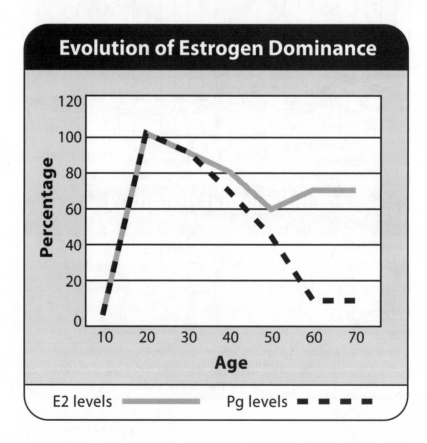

Estrogen Dominance

John Lee, MD, a pioneer in the field of hormone balancing, described the shift toward too much estrogen as "estrogen dominance." Back in the early 70s, Dr. Lee discovered that most women were functionally low in progesterone. He stumbled across this discovery while looking for treatment alternatives to estrogen for his breast cancer patients with osteoporosis. Because excess estrogen can actually promote breast cancer, it is a risky treatment option for cancer survivors, forcing him to look deeper for a substitute.

Though incidental, Dr. Lee's discovery was more science than luck. He understood that women's progesterone production declined more rapidly than estrogen production and that essentially all women in their late 30s become estrogen dominant in relationship to progesterone. At the time, doctors were prescribing estrogen for menopausal women, further exacerbating this estrogen imbalance. As years of estrogen replacement therapy passed, breast and endometrial cancers rose, and most of the conventional medical world did not quickly make the link between estrogen and cancer.

Because he didn't want to give estrogen to his patients with osteoporosis, he turned to transdermal progesterone, a hormone he knew to be beneficial in building bone. He observed that not only did these women have increased bone mineralization and reversed osteoporosis, they experienced relief from a host of PMS and menopausal symptoms. Serendipitously, science, intuition, and trial and error yielded a new understanding of how a woman's hormones worked, and more importantly, a new treatment approach for optimizing hormone balance was born.

To his credit, Dr. Lee took his cue from clinical observation, watching his patients' symptoms improve by supplementing with progesterone. Curiously, however, the rise in progesterone levels could not be substantiated though blood tests, yet the benefit to patients was obvious. It was only years later after developing saliva testing that Dr. Lee could confirm his hunch. He found that women using transdermal progesterone had similar or much higher progesterone (Pg) to estrogen (E2) ratios in their saliva tests when compared with the balance found in younger, healthier women. Conversely, women without sufficient progesterone production had lower Pg/E2 ratios, or estrogen dominance. His simple, yet profound, empirical observations have since been confirmed by a number of medical studies, as well as in clinical practice, including our own.[20–22]

Estrogen dominance essentially impacts every woman at some point in her menstrual lifecycle, but the level of imbalance varies depending upon genetic makeup, nutrition, exposure to environmental toxins, and emotional stressors. Estrogen dominance is important to recognize because it not only leads to many of the symptoms women experience during the later years of their menstrual cycles, it also contributes to bone calcium loss, increases the risk of breast and uterine cancer, and affects brain function, emotional stability, energy level, libido, and sleep.[23]

What About Iodine Deficiency, Estrogen Dominance, and Thyroid Function?

Balancing the progesterone to estrogen ratio with bioidentical progesterone can reverse most common perimenopausal and menopausal symptoms—including those associated with premenstrual syndrome (PMS). However, it is important to acknowledge a backroom player in the development of estrogen dominance. The association of iodine levels, estrogen, and breast tissue changes have been in the literature for over 30 years. Iodine is required for normal breast function. Iodine studies done using rodents demonstrate that iodine deficiency leads to changes in estrogen receptors that lead to enhanced proliferation of breast tissue. These changes are associated with a progression from normal breast tissue to fibrocystic changes to atypia (slightly abnormal cells) to dysplasia (precancerous cells) to neoplasia (cancer).[24] Breast tissue actually competes for iodine stores with the thyroid gland.

According to the World Health Organization, 15 percent of American women are iodine deficient and one third of the world's population is iodine deficient.[25] An even greater number of Americans are marginally iodine sufficient. The recommended daily allowance (RDA) of iodine in the United States is 150 *micro*grams, a small fraction of the 13.8 *milli*grams consumed in mainland Japan, where hypothyroidism and breast cancer is much less common.[26] The U.S. RDA was determined as the amount needed to prevent goiter (enlarged thyroid gland) and cretinism (severe hypothyroidism with mental retardations), not minimize risk of hormone-dependent cancers or optimize our thyroid hormone production. This helps explain why women have a six to ten times higher incidence of low thyroid hormone production, and why it often begins showing up at puberty, when estrogen dependent breasts begin to develop.[27]

The World Around Us: Environmental Toxins

Environmental pollutants affect virtually everyone on the planet every day. We all breathe air polluted with gas and diesel fuel exhaust particles, drink water contaminated by pesticides and herbicides, and eat food that has been exposed to pesticides and herbicides or injected with antibiotics and hormones. Exposure is even worse for people who live in developing countries where pollution is less regulated. We are now seeing the long-term affects of pesticide, herbicide, and hormone additive overuse. The motto made famous in the 50s, "better living through chemistry," has come back to haunt us.

Environmental toxins, including heavy metals, cause imbalances to the endocrine system, which directly affects hormone production. These intolerances are now linked to many major illnesses ranging from cancer to neurodegenerative diseases like Alzheimer's, to autism and attention deficit disorder (ADD), to infertility.[28-34] The current breast cancer and autism epidemics can be directly correlated with increased levels of pollutants in our food, air, and water.[35-38] Even infant umbilical cord blood and breast milk now carry high levels of these toxic chemicals.[39-40]

The group of environmental toxins most responsible for causing health problems is generally known as persistent organic pollutants (POPs). The most common of which, organochlorine compounds, harmfully accumulate in the air, water, and food chains. In humans, organochlorine compounds are stored in body fat where they can sit for decades. Western cultures, particularly those in the Americas, are exposed to 15,000 different organochlorines during a lifetime.[41]

Xenoestrogens

Particularly significant among these pollutants are xenohormones, which once they have penetrated our bodies mimic our natural hormones. They are chemically similar enough to natural hormones that they trick the recognition sites (receptors) on our cells' surface membranes. Because most xenohormones have an estrogen-like effect, they are often referred to as xenoestrogens (XEs).

As a class of human-made chemicals, xenoestrogens are derived from pesticides, herbicides, and fertilizers whose compounds mimic some of estrogen's actions in the body. We know they are pervasive in women's systems, because they are found in breast milk and fetal umbilical cord blood.[42,43] Further evidence shows breast cancer and retarded neurological development have definitively been associated with these compounds, a phenomenon that has been known, but ignored, for decades.[44-48] Though not the most toxic, DDT and dioxins are the XEs most of us are familiar with due to news media coverage.

XEs appear to be playing an increasingly significant role in menstruating women's tendency toward estrogen dominance. Knowing that research has linked breast cancer to excess estrogen relative to progesterone, and that XEs act as additional estrogen in our systems, a direct connection, assuming exposure, is evident. The message estrogen relays is, "Initiate cell growth." Increased levels of XEs in our bodies can be directly correlated to the significant increase in breast, ovarian, and prostate cancer in the United States and other industrialized nations.[49-52]

Nutritional Choices Can Minimize Exposure

We are exposed to POPs and heavy metals through the water supply, and dairy product, meat, and fish consumption. You can minimize your exposure to XEs by carefully choosing what you consume. Eat organic fruits and vegetables, hormone-free meats, and minimally processed foods. Drink filtered or purified water. There is overwhelming evidence that an organic plant-based, low-fat diet is your best defense against environmental toxins.[53]

You can also rid your body of these toxins through various detoxification treatments, which we recommend doing under the guidance of a qualified health care professional (*see* "Appendix A: Resources & Tools: Stacking the Deck").

◄ 3 ►
What Are Your Hormones Doing?

Fluctuating hormones have many faces. Menopause and its onset phase, perimenopause, arrive in different ways for different women. Most women, at some point, have hot flashes or night sweats, but there is a wide spectrum of intensity and frequency of even these symptoms. Symptoms are as varied and unique as individuals. What you can count on is that hormone swings will likely exacerbate your existing health issues or weaknesses. If, for example, you have always had a tendency to be anxious or depressed, you will probably experience longer and more intense episodes as you enter mid-life. Or if you have had blood sugar issues such as hypoglycemia, it will likely be exaggerated by hormonal changes. This comes as no surprise to those of you who are already in the midst of mid-life hormonal shifts. If you are just beginning the journey, you fortunately may be able to avoid the symptoms of extreme hormone swings by keeping them or getting them back in balance early on.

Specific signs and symptoms can be broken up into three general areas: physical, emotional, and mental. Below you will find descriptions of some of the most common symptoms within each of these areas. Keep in mind that there can be multiple causes of these symptoms; not all of them are necessarily hormone related.

At the end of this chapter, we have provided a "Hormone Imbalance Pretest" for you to take to get a rough idea of your particular hormone picture. Once you determine your score, you can read more on the characteristics of that imbalance. While you may feel certain about your particular hormone imbalance after reading about the symptoms and taking the pretest, getting a lab test and finding a practitioner to support you through this transitional time is the only way to be sure your assessment is accurate. Remember, whatever your symptoms, take heart, there is help and hope ahead.

Signs and Symptoms

Typical Signs of Hormone Imbalance

- weight gain
- decreased or no sex drive
- hot flashes/night sweats
- migraine headaches
- insomnia
- fatigue
- anxiety/panic
- depression
- low self-esteem
- emotional fragility
- irritability
- anger
- brain fog
- forgetfulness
- hypercritical and obsessive thinking

Weight Gain: Extra Pounds Getting You Down?

Weight gain is the most common complaint we hear about in initial visits with patients. In fact, it is a tremendous problem for the population at large. According to the Centers for Disease Control, obesity has reached epidemic proportions in the United States.[54] There are many contributing factors fueling this trend, none more important than the slowing of our metabolic rate as we age.

We have patients who diet, exercise, and eat the right foods and still gain weight or can't lose the extra pounds that have slowly accumulated around their mid-section, thighs, and hips. Aside from cosmetic consequences, weight gain creates an extra burden on the pancreas to control blood sugars in a healthy range, leading to the explosion of diabetes in adults as well as children in this country. The consequences of adult-onset diabetes can be catastrophic: kidney failure, blindness, heart disease, and stroke. In any case, maintaining a healthy weight is an aim worth your ongoing effort. It is not an exaggeration to say that getting your weight under control could save your life.

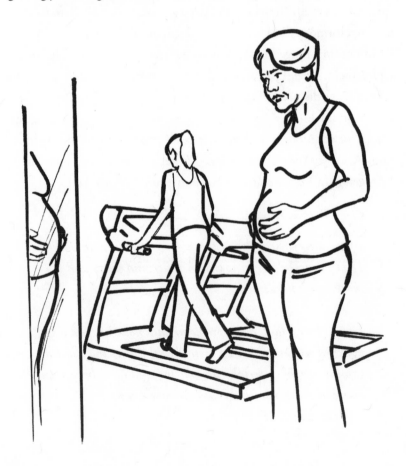

Hormone deficiencies can play a significant role in weight gain. This includes imbalances in thyroid, progesterone, estrogen, and cortisol, among others. Estrogen and progesterone imbalances are particularly common, along with cortisol over or underproduction and androgen (testosterone and DHEA) imbalances. Correcting hormonal excesses or deficiencies will often have a major impact on correcting blood sugar elevations, while also improving lean body mass (proportion of fat to muscle).

Low thyroid levels can cause weight gain. What your physician may not realize is that the current standard criterion for evaluating thyroid function is flawed. The laboratory criterion for abnormal Thyroid Stimulating Hormone (TSH) is too broad.[55] Some TSH levels identified as within normal range should actually be treated with thyroid hormone replacement. Even if you previously have had your thyroid checked and been told it's disease-free, it doesn't necessarily mean your thyroid levels are optimal. (*See* "Appendix A: Resources & Tools: Stacking the Deck" for additional recommended reading on optimal thyroid function. Also, see iodine discussion, "What About Iodine Deficiency, Estrogen Dominance, and Thyroid Function?" on page 46.)

I have always struggled with weight gain, but nothing like I am now. The weight comes on easier and faster and it is much, much harder to lose.

I have never had a weight problem, until now. I have always exercised regularly, eaten a pretty healthy diet, and I'm still gaining weight, especially around my middle. I have even been exercising more and eating less to stop the gain. Nothing seems to matter. The pounds seem to be here to stay.

Decreased or No Sex Drive: Sex on the Back Burner?

When working with patients, we often ask two questions regarding sexual experience: How is your libido or interest in sex and has it changed?, and, How well does your body respond to sexual stimulation? While some women may lose their libido, they find that when and if sexually active their bodies are still very responsive and able to reach orgasm. Other women will experience a slowing of their physical responsiveness. It takes a great deal more time to reach orgasm, or they may report that they simply do not attain orgasm anymore.

All the sex hormones play a role in sexual arousal and responsiveness or libido. As we age, loss of libido is a common complaint of both men and women. There have been many claims in the media that testosterone will cause your sex drive to return. But less than half of women

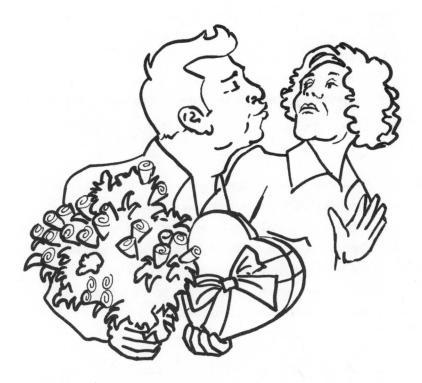

recover their libido through testosterone therapy. For most women with diminished sex drive, deficient testosterone levels is not the only problem. Women vary in the extent to which testosterone levels affect their libido.

When a testosterone deficiency is not an obvious cause, other hormone imbalances or deficiencies or both must be explored. More often low sex drive is a combination of several hormone changes influencing sexual drive and responsiveness. This can include estrogen to progesterone imbalance, low thyroid hormone levels, or adrenal gland over- or underproduction. These multidimensional hormone influences help explain why women's sexual responsiveness is so powerfully influenced by mood, energy, well-being, and other psychological mechanisms. When returned to pre-perimenopausal levels, estrogen increases vaginal blood flow, helping to restore the vaginal lining and increase lubrication and elasticity of the vaginal column; progesterone may help with uplifting mood factors that impact sexual response; and testosterone enhances mood and energy. Sometimes it takes a little time and tweaking, but once the right balance of hormones is accomplished most women experience renewed sexual vitality.

My sex drive when I was younger was pretty good. I had friends who seemed more energized than I did that way, yet I felt good and satisfied sexually. Now I'm dead that way. Seriously, I have no interest whatsoever, and if I am sexual, it feels like a lot of work—too much effort. I try to accommodate my husband every once in awhile, but he's not that interested either knowing I'm not into it.

Hot Flashes and Night Sweats:
Is It Hot in Here or Is It Just Me?

If someone knows nothing else about perimenopause or menopause, they know about hot flashes. If you have experienced them first hand, you know what it's like to wake up drenched in sweat or suddenly become so flushed you think you could explode or burst into flames? Night sweats and hot flashes are among the most common symptoms reported by our patients. They can be debilitating or simply a mild inconvenience. The variability of their intensity and frequency is as varied as the fingerprints of the women reporting them.

Hot flashes are the result of blood vessel instability due to fluctuations in estrogen, progesterone, or testosterone, or any combination of the three. Although the exact mechanism of the vasomotor instability is not known, the association with hormone imbalance is very clear. Symptoms are readily corrected by balancing hormones with the right bioidentical replacements.

———————————

The fortunate woman:

> *It's no big deal. I don't know what women are making such a fuss about.*

The unfortunate woman:

> *I'm not myself anymore. I wake up every night three to four times, often drenched in sweat. In the morning, I feel more tired than when I went to bed. At work, I have even had to leave a business meeting because I was so uncomfortable and embarrassed. You can actually see the hot flashes; my face turns beet red!*

———————————

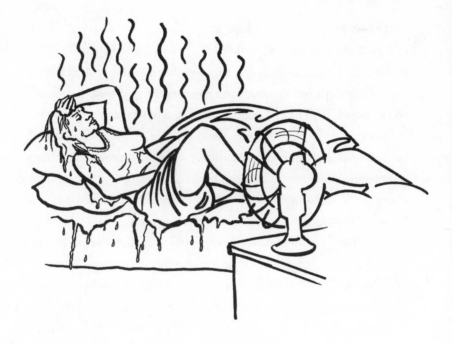

Insomnia: Wide Awake at 4:00 a.m.?

Do you have trouble getting to sleep or do you wake up several times
a night and then have difficulty getting back to sleep? Before you rush
out and buy the latest and greatest sleeping pill, consider the hormone
imbalance connection, adrenal gland under- or overproduction, or a
neurotransmitter or melatonin deficiency. A pill may help you sleep,
but it will not correct the problem. Sorting out the exact imbalance
or deficiency may involve some testing. But when hormones are the
problem, achieving the right balance of estrogen and progesterone levels can restore normal sleep patterns. Because disrupted sleep patterns
can involve many factors, treatment may require several related natural
therapies. When taking this approach, patients rarely have to resort to
a pharmaceutical remedy.

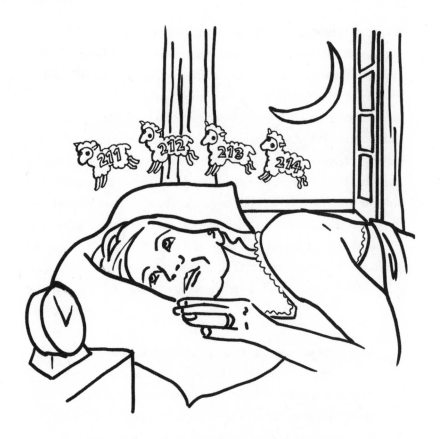

I used to sleep soundly every night from the time I laid down until my alarm clock rang in the morning. Now, the past three to four months, I drop into bed each night exhausted, and my limbs are heavy with fatigue. I'll fall asleep only to wake up one or two hours later. And wide-awake I will stay—often for three or four hours—I mean really awake. Then about the time I need to get up, I finally start to feel sleepy again.

Migraine Headaches: Ready to Divorce Your Head?

Like hot flashes, migraine headaches are caused by vascular instability, primarily blood vessels in the brain. The exact mechanism of blood instability, as with hot flashes, is not known, and it varies between individuals. For some it is due to blood vessels that dilate inappropriately, and in others it is due to blood vessels that constrict inappropriately. Having opposite causes explains why sometimes pharmaceuticals work and other times they are ineffective. By design they are created to treat only the vasodilatation form of migraine. There are several theories on the cause: allergies, mineral deficiencies, stress, hormone imbalance, and more. In our experience, approximately 50 percent of migraine headaches in women are cyclical, related to menstruation. They are thus most often correctable by rebalancing estrogen and progesterone.

As a younger woman, I came to expect my monthly migraines. They came like clockwork not unlike my regular 28-day menstrual cycle. The headaches would last a day or two and that would be it until the next month. I even had nine months in a row of no migraines; both times I was pregnant with my children. Then perimenopause struck, and now I can have anywhere from 5–20 days of migraine headache a month. I am still getting my periods—albeit erratic and irregular now—but the migraines have started to dominate my life. I've even had times when I've wondered whether or not I can keep my job because I'm getting so many migraines. Sometimes the medication I take doesn't help and I have to go home and lie in a dark room.

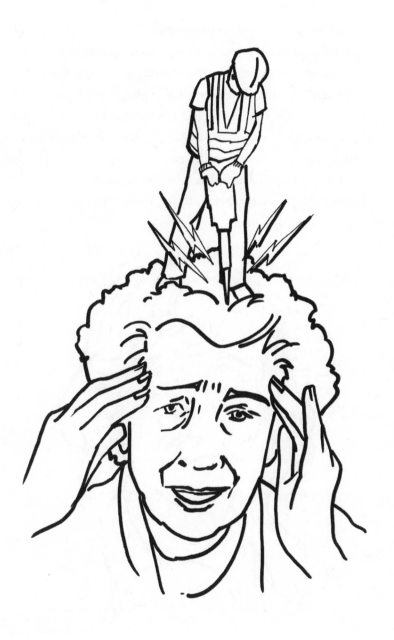

Fatigue: Exhausted All of the Time?

Fatigue is an extremely common complaint in midlife and beyond. It often is exasperating and worrisome when you have experienced vitality most of your life, to suddenly feel unplugged. Because there are often many contributing factors like low thyroid, poor adrenal gland function, and sex hormone imbalances, it may take a few visits and thorough testing to ferret out the cause(s). Each possible cause and how to correct the problem will be discussed in detail in Chapter 5. Fatigue is one the most reversible of all symptoms using natural remedies and bioidentical hormones.

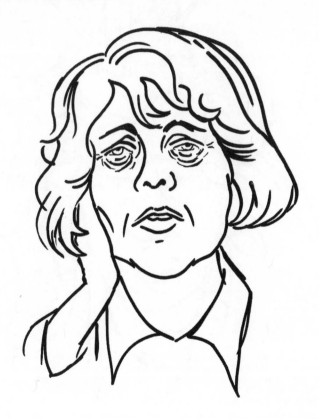

I've always been an energetic person, but lately I'm noticing that I feel tired all the time, even mid-morning when I've only been awake for a few hours. Since I started menopausing, I have been slowing down. It's getting to the point where I don't have the energy to exercise anymore, and I do nothing in the evenings after work. I can just plop down on the couch after making a microwave popcorn, turn on TV, and not rise again until bedtime! That is so not me. I used to go out and do things or work on projects at home, but I feel too tired now.

Riding The Emotional Rollercoaster

Many women are surprised to learn that mid-life hormone shifts often come with pronounced emotional side effects such as anxiety, depression, and emotional fragility. Hormonal balance plays a significant role in modulating and modifying our emotional responses. The specific players are the same five we have been talking about: sex hormones (estrogen, progesterone, and testosterone); adrenal hormones (cortisol and DHEA); and neurotransmitters (norepinephrine and epinephrine) produced along with cortisol and DHEA in the adrenal glands.

As you enter perimenopause you begin producing less progesterone, throwing off your normal estrogen/progesterone ratios. At the same time, your estrogen levels can fluctuate drastically swinging you into states of estrogen dominance. While every woman reacts to estrogen dominance differently, common mental and emotional effects include fatigue, irritability, inability to handle stress, depression, anxiety, and mood swings, among other physical symptoms already discussed.

Anxiety & Panic: Suddenly Fearing Fear Itself?

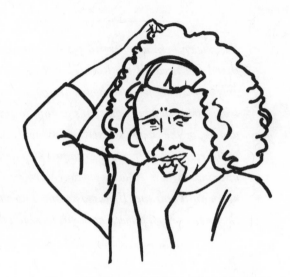

Most women do not realize that anxiety can be brought on by hormonal imbalances. So often patients tell us that until their late 40s they had never experienced an anxiety attack. Yet as they enter mid-life, anxiety has become a chronic problem. Some women report having had some anxiety during young adulthood but nothing compared with the anxiety they are currently experiencing now in mid-life.

Your propensity for anxiety prior to perimenopause may be compounded once your menopausal transition begins. Imagine after experiencing significant stress during your early childhood years, you then take another hit at puberty when your body rapidly goes into major sex hormone production, which, like the early stress, takes its toll on your adrenal glands. You then go on to lead a stressful lifestyle for many years, also adding to the stress load on your adrenal glands. Finally, when you arrive at middle age and your hormonal system begins to wane, you require more work from your adrenal glands to make up for the lower levels of sex hormones. Your depleted adrenal glands don't have the reserves after being doubly or triply stressed over your lifetime to take up the slack. Years of overused adrenal glands are a sure invitation for anxiety and panic to rear their ugly heads. It is no wonder panic attacks or anxiety disorders often come with menopause.

I awoke suddenly in the middle of the night with my heart beating fast and hard. I lay frozen in my dark room, intently listening for the source of the danger that had surely roused me. It would have been an appropriate response had someone been breaking into my home, but the house was perfectly still. I got out of bed and made a room-by-room check of the house. All was quiet and secure. Yet, the terror in my chest would not ease. This was the third wakeful night in a row. I would spend another night wide-awake, waiting out the psychological storm, somehow trusting sanity would return. I knew I could get through another sleepless night, but underneath it all, I had begun to wonder if I was going crazy. Day and night, new fears had begun to crowd my thoughts. I had a constant sense of impending doom and often daydreamed about worst-case scenarios.

It wasn't until six months later that I got a glimpse of a possible cause. Up to that point, I was still having three to four sleepless nights a week, and dragging myself out of bed each morning, feeling like I was losing ground each day. But on this particular night, I was again awakened by the feelings of terror in my chest, my heart thudding like the marching band's base drum. Only this time, I was very hot and even slightly sweaty. The heat wave lasted two or three minutes, and then I was cold enough to want all the blankets on again. This must be a hot flash or night sweats, I thought. Was this the beginning of menopause, I asked myself?

Depression: Feeling Down and Don't Know Why?

For some, depression peeks around the corner and taunts them occasionally; for others, it smacks them in the face and knocks them off their feet. In perimenopause and menopause, we observe clinically that prior mood issues can, for some, be exacerbated by hormonal disruption. Imbalanced hormones alone can create mood disturbances. Sometimes this mood disruption is heralded by short-temperedness and irritability, other times, a resignation about life and all that was once engaging becomes eroded by the loss of vitality and optimal hormone levels.

In our clinic we have seen many women who report neither prior mood difficulties nor battles with previous depression. They often say it hits them out of the blue with comments like, "I just quit caring about

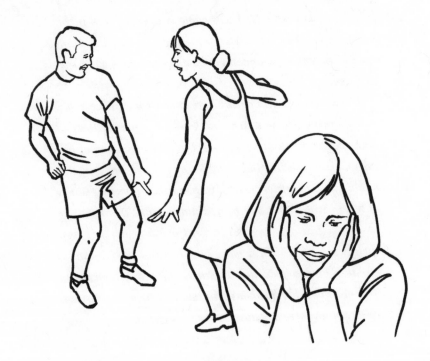

everything . . . about life," and "all the things I used to be involved in at home and at work are burdens or not interesting to me now."

Many times mothers hit their perimenopausal phase of life at the same time their children are leaving home (empty nest syndrome), and their aging parents require assistance. A patient recently shared that not only did her last child leave home this fall, but her mother died, and her father needed to be cared for through assisted living or by moving in with them. In addition, she was not sleeping due to hot flashes and night sweats, and her libido was completely gone. No wonder she felt depressed. Despite this patient's outer life challenges, rebalancing her hormones will go a long way in helping her handle the multiple and challenging life events.

Symptoms of Depression

- loss of interest and enjoyment of your favorite activities
- sadness
- fatigue
- sleep disturbance (too much or too little)
- changes in appetite
- difficulty concentrating
- aches and pains
- excessive and inappropriate feelings of guilt
- thoughts of death and suicide
- difficulty making decisions
- feelings of worthlessness

Since the onset of puberty, I have struggled with depression. I have gone on and off antidepressants, but for the most part, have managed a fairly normal, functional life. But things seemed to take a turn for the worse over the past few years. I am 46 now and have begun to wonder if melancholy is going to finally overtake me. What used to be a subtle, underlying sadness is now, at times, an overwhelming feeling of gloom and doom. It doesn't make sense. Nothing has changed. I still have a good marriage, two healthy, well-adjusted children, and a job that I enjoy. Yet the depression is worse than ever and it feels like I'm losing ground every day.

Low Self-Esteem: Confidence Out the Window?

When we talk about feelings of low self-esteem in this context, it is a narrow definition, episodic, not necessarily a life-long issue. Women who are going through hormonal transitions often report inexplicable and instantaneous shifts in their feelings of self worth. These feelings can be powerful, overwhelming, and seemingly without cause.

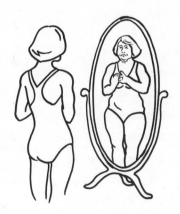

I thought I'd left that sophomoric fear about what other people think of me back in high school, or at least in my 20s. Hadn't I paid thousands of dollars and spent countless hours in therapy to build a new, better me? Or at least to learn how to respect and love the person I am? Where now was all of that quiet self-confidence I fought so hard to build? Wasn't I an accomplished professional and a good mother? For all the self-esteem I've been able to muster lately, I feel more like a pimply-faced teenager than a self-assured, middle-aged woman. What happened?

Emotional Fragility: Feel Like You're Falling Apart?

Women who report emotional fragility describe a volatile state in which they feel like their world is coming apart at the seams. They may be assertive and pragmatic one day and wake up the next feeling barely able to keep from sobbing about the weather. Nothing has changed but their hormone levels, particularly progesterone.

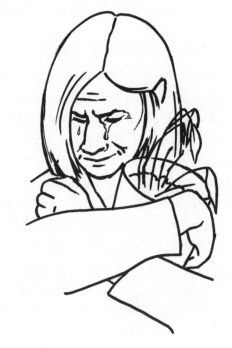

I cry over television commercials, greeting cards, news stories, and for that matter, spilled milk. I am a yo-yo of emotions. Unkind remarks that used to roll off of my back now feel like mortal wounds. One minute I'm laughing hysterically, the next I'm sobbing uncontrollably or spinning out in worry and fear. I never used to be like this. Oh I had the occasional weepy day right around my period, but other than that, I have always been the one with the cool head and the even temper. Not anymore. I try hard to hide it, but inside it's like I'm falling apart. I hate how out of control I feel. I often wonder if I'm losing my mind. What if I am truly hysterical? How long before people at work start thinking I'm unprofessional, or even incompetent? I am desperate to get back to firmer ground. I just want my old self back!

Irritability & Anger: Blowing Up Without Notice?

Those of you who have suffered from PMS know irritability is a part of hormonal shifts. Unfortunately, however, as you go through menopause that same PMS period generally lasts longer and is, in many cases, more intense than during earlier phases of your life. It is not uncommon to hear women talk about having less impulse control, losing their tempers more easily, and feeling startled and frustrated by the power of their reactions.

Also, it is not uncommon to experience strain within your family. You may feel isolated as your spouse or children begin avoiding you because you may fly off the handle or lose it at the least provocation. It is discouraging to notice that in years past situations where you had been caring, understanding, and compassionate now leave you feeling

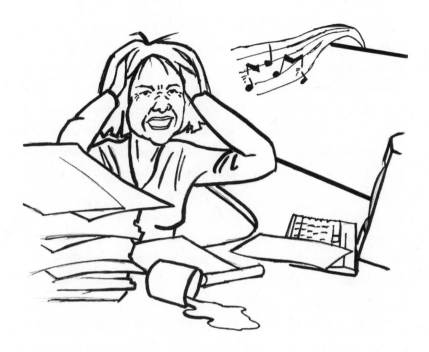

inconvenienced and overwhelmed. Know that correcting your hormone imbalances can lead you back into the good graces of family and friends.

I have always been a pretty even-keeled person—never getting too upset or distraught emotionally—but lately, man, don't get in my way 'cause I'm dangerous when annoyed. And it seems like I'm annoyed a lot of the time. I feel irritated and angry with my partner, I'm more judgmental and critical of people I work with, and I have even been getting angry while driving. This is crazy and not me!

Brain Fog or Forgetfulness:
Wait It Will Come to Me . . . Or Will It?

With the onset of perimenopause, your memory probably works pretty efficiently most of the time, but you may be experiencing lapses in what you can remember. Memory loss is a natural part of aging. But menopausal women often complain of brain fog or the inability to retrieve certain information when they need it. This is usually information you know, but it stubbornly doesn't come at the moment you are trying to recall it.

Estrogen fluctuations occurring during menopause have long been blamed for these reported cognitive lapses. Estrogen stimulates neurotransmitters that allow parts of your brain to communicate with one another. It also helps dilate blood vessels in the brain, increasing the flow of red blood cells that help the brain to function. However, stress and sleep disruptions may play substantial roles in these cogni-

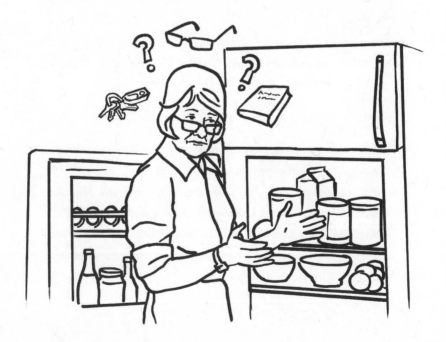

tive complaints as well. So it is estrogen, but it is also neurotransmitter activity, adrenal health, and a woman's experience of insomnia, all of which help explain why this is a time when memory and mental challenges flourish.

I walked into my office one day and discovered a beautiful bouquet of flowers on my desk with no note. A co-worker and friend happened to stop by my office, and we both mused over who could have sent the flowers. We were interrupted by a phone call, my friend left my office, and I went back to work. A half hour later, after completely blanking out our conversation, I called my friend to tell her that someone had sent me flowers and did she have any idea who?

"Sarah," she reminded me, *"I was* THERE *when you found the flowers, remember?" I stopped, horrified. I knew she was right, but I honestly couldn't connect that knowledge with the memory. We made a joke and moved on. I eventually remembered, but was deeply shaken. What had happened to my sharp, nimble mind? Was this the first stage of Alzheimer's or some other neurological disorder?*

And there were other changes besides blanking out entirely; I often couldn't think clearly. Sometimes trying to follow the logic of an argument was like wading through Jell-O. Thoughts came slowly or got derailed altogether. It was like watching a nightmare in slow motion. My mind was the one thing I had always been able to rely on. My quick wit, my strategic insight, my creative flair—all of these things were a huge part of my identity. They were crumbling before my eyes. Where would it end?

Obsessive or Hypercritical Thinking: Troubling Thoughts Running You Ragged?

Another way women can experience mental disturbances from hormone imbalance manifests as difficulty letting go of a bothersome thought. The most responsible hormone is cortisol, produced in the adrenal glands. When triggered into the fight or flight response, our cortisol levels rise and our brains get instructed to memorize the experienced danger or difficulty so we can protect ourselves better if it happens again. This creates a worn pattern; thoughts travel down the same neuronal pathway over and over again even though the trauma has long past.

Prior to getting your period, you can often feel more critical of yourself, even insecure, as in the teenage girl who changes outfits prior to school six times. Clinically, we see this same rattling of self-esteem during perimenopause and menopause. It's no wonder since the ovarian hormones that fluctuate during PMS are again fluctuating as they dramatically decline during perimenopause. When balanced and at functional levels, these hormones directly affect many aspects of your well-being, confidence, and overall disposition.

Week in and week out, we have women admit in our offices that they feel unattractive, or fat and ugly, or dead sexually. We also see a hypercritical thinking trend among these women. They are unable to shut off their critical brain; if something is bothering them, it wears a rut into their thoughts and they can't stop obsessing and worrying about their concerns. Many say these thoughts are driving them crazy or they feel as if they are going crazy.

With this combination of hypercritical and obsessive thinking, whether it's a concern about yourself or something out in the world, perimenopausal hormone imbalances can cause you to over think and fret to the point of tearing yourself to proverbial shreds.

I obsess over the smallest details—things that would never have thrown me in the past. A thoughtless comment by my next-door neighbor, the imagined ways I'm failing my family, my partner's inattention. My mind goes over and over these things like a dog with a bone.

It's as if a switch gets turned on and I hear a running dialogue in my head of all that is wrong—in myself and others. I don't consider myself a hypercritical person, but when my hormones are raging, my inner critic is relentless. It's exhausting!

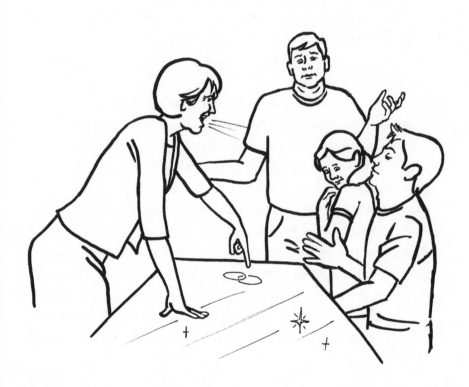

The Serious Consequences of
Untreated Mid-Life Hormone Imbalance

While the symptoms of hormone imbalance can have a profound impact on a woman's day-to-day life, chronic imbalance can play a role in more serious, even life-threatening health conditions. This includes breast, ovarian, and endometrial cancers, heart disease, stroke, diabetes, and osteoporosis.

Breast and Endometrial Cancer

More than 200,000 American women are told they have breast cancer each year. Forty thousand women die from the disease in spite of the fact that $6 billion is spent on research annually.[56] Based on our understanding of human physiology, the research, and our clinical experience using bioidentical hormones the majority of breast cancers could be prevented. In fact, there is overwhelming data showing that the conventional medical approach to women's health is contributing to the problem.

Since the introduction of Premarin (a synthetic form of estrogen made from horse mare's urine) in 1942, the evidence has been overwhelming: estrogen has been associated with an increased risk of breast and endometrial cancer. Two studies looking at estrogen-only hormone replacement therapy further validate the risk of cancer due to estrogen dominance. Of the two, the Million Women Study showed a 30 percent increase in risk for developing breast cancer. A third study, the Puget Sound Study reported a 60 percent increased risk over women who were never exposed to estrogen therapy.[57,58]

In fact, progestins like Provera, are synthetically developed to counter this side effect. Progestins however, only mimic some, but not all, of the functions of progesterone, causing them to impose their own set of detrimental side effects. Provera is now known to increase the risk for breast cancer (29% increase), heart disease (26% increase) and stroke (41% increase), while progesterone has none of these side effects.[59]

We highly recommend all women, particularly those with blood relatives, who have developed breast cancer get tested for estrogen dominance. The problem can be easily and safely remedied with bioidentical progesterone.

Heart Disease and Stroke

According to the U.S. Center for Disease Control and Prevention newsletter, 29% of all deaths in the United States are due to cardiovascular disease.[60] Heart disease is the number one leading cause of death in the United States for both men and women. The risk of heart disease and stroke, of course, increases with age and is directly related to decline in hormone production. In women the decline in progesterone relative to estrogen—the estrogen dominance recipe—is a major factor in the development of clogged blood vessels. Furthermore, conventional hormone replacement therapy (HRT) contributes to the risk of heart disease and stroke. The Women's Health Initiative study was abruptly discontinued when a 26% increase in heart disease and 41% increase in stroke occurred among participants.[61] The offender was Provera, the synthetic progestin used in combination with Premarin, also known as PremPro, the FDA-approved HRT drug used by unsuspecting women for decades. Based on the fact that six million women take this drug (the most prescribed drug in the United States) and the incidence of disease reported in this study, we surmise that an estimated 40,000 women per decade are to some degree seriously harmed, or mortally injured, by taking PremPro.

In contrast to estrogen, biological progesterone protects our heart and blood vessels. Not only does progesterone lower cholesterol, enhance fat burning for energy, and reduce inflammation, all of which protect the heart, the medical literature indicates that there are many other beneficial effects. For example, the Harvard School of Public Health reported that progesterone inhibits smooth muscle proliferation.[62] Smooth muscles are a significant factor affecting arteriosclerotic plaque formation, which compromises blood flow and oxygen to the heart muscle and brain. Another study showed when compared with medroxyprogesterone (the generic name for Provera) in combination with estrogen that bioidentical progesterone increased exercise tolerance in postmenopausal women with known heart disease.[63] Evidence points to good nutrition, regular exercise, and, as needed, balancing your hormones with transdermal (topical) progesterone as the best formula for a healthy heart.

Severe Adrenal Fatigue

Long-term stress can exhaust your adrenal glands' ability to make cortisol, throw your hormones into a tailspin, and cause a condition known as severe adrenal fatigue. Years of adrenal over-activity, or cortisol overproduction, can lead to a number of health conditions: chronic fatigue, fibromyalgia, migraines, and a weak immune system, all of which include cortisol underproduction as an underlying condition. When you have the pedal to the metal, you burn more gas, faster, ultimately leaving your tank empty. Often caffeine and sugar cravings, and addictions are a clue that your body is not able to maintain normal cortisol levels, which leaves you dependent on other sources for an energy boost. Eventually, those won't make up for the deficiency either.

Each adrenal gland has a medulla and a cortex, which are responsible for producing specific hormones. The cortex produces steroid hormones, primarily cortisol and DHEA. It also produces some estrogen, progesterone, and testosterone at the point when the ovaries stop producing eggs. The medulla produces epinephrine and adrenalin, the fight or flight hormones. With adrenal fatigue, we are concerned with cortisol production, because it is the master hormone related to energy levels and blood sugar metabolism. Cortisol is essential to life, particularly vitality. If we lose cortisol production completely, we experience a collapse of our cardiovascular system—our heart will literally stop.

Low cortisol levels in perimenopausal and menopausal women with a history of unhealthy stressors can be traced to the intimate connection between progesterone and cortisol production in the body. Progesterone is made from a precursor called pregnenolone. This substance is also the precursor needed to make cortisol and DHEA. Because the body uses hormones based on its own hierarchy of needs, the adrenal glands will demand that the pregnenolone be made into adrenal hormones before being used to make progesterone. The body always chooses survival over reproduction.

Already low in cortisol and DHEA, the menstrual cycle of an unnaturally stressed woman will be compromised by a decrease in progesterone production. If this imbalance begins early in a woman's hormone cycle, she will be headed for a lifetime of progesterone/estrogen imbalance. Estrogen will dominate. This is a sure formula for premenstrual syndrome (PMS), uterine fibroids, ovarian cysts, endometriosis, fibrocystic breasts, and irregular bleeding. As the periods cycle and months add up to years, these conditions can also alter other organ functions, causing what preventive-minded doctors term functional illness. Even if other serious health conditions don't develop a woman will enter midlife with a depleted supply of progesterone. Then due to trauma or simply a high stress lifestyle, the transition into menopause will be further intensified, because there will be no progesterone cushion for the transition.

To correct the problem, cortisol levels must be optimized. Cortisol optimization is an area where conventional medicine has failed patients. Many of us were taught in traditional medical school that patients are either in complete adrenal failure or normal. As with all hormone-producing systems there are shades of gray. Many of our patients report their chief complaint as fatigue, and in fact, about 70 percent of our patient's cortisol level tests turn out to be adequate but not optimal. They are not, yet, in a disease state, but show levels that compromise well-being.

The test used to determine cortisol levels is called a salivary adrenal function test. This test indicates adrenal fatigue when the cortisol graph shows a flat or level line of cortisol throughout a day as opposed to a healthy high morning level that trails off throughout the day. When we see a flattened diurnal curve and corresponding symptoms, we diagnose adrenal gland fatigue. Adrenal fatigue is remedied by supplementing with cortisol, providing nutrients to rebuild adrenal gland function, and addressing lifestyle changes to decrease stress as needed.

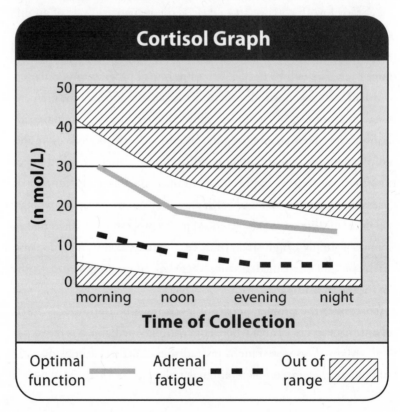

Diabetes

It is now estimated that one in every three Americans will develop Type 2, or adult-onset diabetes in their lifetime. Health officials and doctors place the blame for the rising incidence of Type 2 diabetes on being overweight or obese.[64] Adult onset diabetes diagnosis is occurring more rapidly in children now than in adults, making "adult onset" a misnomer. According to the Centers for Disease Control and Prevention, obesity has more than doubled for preschool children aged 2 to 5 years of age and adolescents aged 12 to 19 since the 1970s. It has more than tripled for children aged 6 to 11 years old.[65] This translates to approximately nine million children over six years of age being obese.

High blood sugar levels have dire consequences for many organs, but none more important than the blood vessels. When sugar levels are high, they interact with the blood vessel wall causing the wall to thicken. If uncontrolled, eventually the blood vessel channel becomes too small to carry sufficient oxygen and other nutrients to vital organs, as in the retina, or light-sensing layer in our eyes, kidneys, heart, brain, and limbs. Most of us know someone who has had a stroke, heart attack, lost vision, or required an amputation or kidney transplant as a direct result of diabetes.

Type 2 diabetes is a disease caused by hormone imbalances and it doesn't happen overnight. There are many warning signs along the way. So many, in fact, that a separate pre-diabetic condition has been identified. The most popular current term for this is metabolic syndrome. Other terms used are insulin resistance and syndrome X. Insulin resistance actually best describes the condition because of the strong connection between obesity and diabetes.

While neither insulin resistance nor diabetes is directly linked to perimenopause or menopause, the connection comes with women's tendency toward weight gain as their progesterone levels drop. Normal progesterone levels help inhibit the formation of fat. Women entering menopause who have not or do not exercise regularly, haven't

or don't eat a healthy diet, or have a history of excessive stress are particularly vulnerable to this side effect of deficient progesterone. Drops
in progesterone and occasionally testosterone levels cause fat to collect around our midsections, belly, and intestines. Unlike other fat,
this particular kind of fat requires more insulin to push the sugar into
cells. If the pancreas has to work overtime for too long, it will eventually fail to balance blood sugar, allowing it to rise unchecked throughout the body. Furthermore, excess insulin alone leads to blood vessel
disease. Elevated insulin (hyperinsulinism) is creating a disease state
long before blood sugar levels are high.

You know, or might imagine, the rest of the story. Insulin resistance
and diabetes are a real concern for perimenopausal and menopausal
women, particularly if they have any other risk factors. The good news
is, if you heed the warning signs—triglyceride and insulin elevations,
and low progesterone levels—insulin resistance is completely reversible with diet, exercise changes, and bioidentical hormone replacement
therapy to correct progesterone deficiency. If you are concerned about
whether your insulin resistance is part of your hormone imbalance picture, be sure to discuss this with your doctor.

Osteoporosis: The Bare Bones Truth

At age 30, your bones reach their peak of strength. After this peak,
they gradually become less dense, increasing the risk for developing
osteoporosis, a condition of porous bones, which are more fragile and
prone to breaking. Mineral and vitamin deficiencies; corticosteroid
drugs like cortisone; poor eating habits (eating excess dairy and meat,
and drinking soda pop); smoking; lack of weight-bearing exercise; too
much cortisol; and too little estrogen, progesterone, and testosterone
are all contributing causes of osteoporosis. Osteoporosis affects 44
million Americans, 80 percent of whom are female.[66]

While there are multiple factors leading to osteoporosis, hormones play a significant role. Estrogen regulates the activity of the osteoclasts. These are bone-preservers that slow the process of older bone dissolution. Progesterone and testosterone regulate the activity of osteoblasts, which affect the formation of new bone. Estrogen can temporarily slow down but it cannot reverse osteoporosis, and it cannot protect against osteoporosis at all when progesterone is absent. It appears that only natural ovarian-secreted or bioidentical progesterone and testosterone are capable of reversing the osteoporosis process by initiating increased numbers of osteoblasts to rebuild bone. Prevention through diet, lifestyle choices, and natural hormone balancing can prevent you from developing osteoporosis.

Hormone Balance Pretest

To get a better idea of your hormone balance status, you can begin by identifying and classifying your symptoms. The following test will help you determine whether your symptoms are the result of an imbalance along with what type of imbalance it is.

Rate the following symptoms from 0–3:
0 = no experience; 1 = slight or occasional experience; 2 = moderate or common experience; 3 = severe or frequent experience

Symptoms	0	1	2	3
A				
Hot flashes				
Night sweats				
Vaginal dryness				
Increased forgetfulness				
Foggy thinking				
Tearfulness				
Mood swings				

Symptoms	0	1	2	3
B				
Tender breasts				
Menstrual bleeding changes				
Uterine fibroids or ovarian cysts				
Water retention or bloating				
Depression				
Anxiety				
Moodiness				
C				
Acne				
Unwanted hair growth				
Scalp hair loss				
Increased sweating				
Short tempered				
High blood sugar				
Weight gain around middle				
D				
Morning fatigue				
Stress				
Difficulty sleeping				
Diminishing stamina				
Irritability				
Extreme alarm/startle response				
Sugar cravings				
Cold hands and feet				
Frequent low level headaches and slight feeling of nausea				
E				
Dizzy spells				
High cholesterol				

Constipation				
Brittle and breaking nails				
Dry skin				
Hair dryness, breakage, loss				
Swelling of eyes and face				
F				
Decreased sweating				
Decreased libido				
Allergy				
Decreased muscle size and strength				
Aches and pains				
Bone loss				
G				
Fibromyalgia				
Rapid aging				
Thinning skin				
Hearing loss				
Fatigue				
Joint and muscle pain				
Overall lack of vitality				
TOTALS				

Key:

A = Estrogen deficiency

B = Estrogen dominance with progesterone deficiency

C = Adrenal fatigue

D = High blood sugar with insulin resistance

E = Low metabolism and subclinical hypothyroidism

F = Testosterone deficiency

G = Human growth hormone deficiency

Interpreting Your Scores

If you scored 6–21 points in any individual section, you likely have an established hormone imbalance in that area. If you scored 1–5 points in any section, your hormones may still be headed toward imbalance. In either case you can reverse the condition or trend with bioidentical hormone replacement therapy and better lifestyle choices. Following are explanations of each type of hormone imbalance as it is categorized in the Hormone Pretest sections A-G.

A. Estrogen Deficiency

A high score in this category may mean you are deficient in estrogen, but this diagnosis can be misleading. Most doctors are trained to see classic menopausal symptoms like hot flashes, night sweats, and mood swings as symptoms of low estrogen, no questions asked. Too often estrogen deficiency is the blanket diagnosis. While only about 20 percent of women are actually estrogen deficient, most conventionally trained MDs assume women's symptoms are caused by low estrogen and will prescribe a non-bioidentical estrogen (HRT) to raise levels without testing or accurately assessing all sex hormone levels.

In fact, most women with symptoms of estrogen deficiency early in menopause are actually experiencing a dynamic dance between estrogen and progesterone, a transition that involves erratic fluctuations in estrogen (highs and lows) and a simultaneous plummeting of progesterone levels (see discussion below on high estrogen). It is during this transition that symptoms are the most profound and bothersome. The key to determining whether you simply have low estrogen, or are in the midst of a dynamic fluctuation between estrogen and progesterone, will be to do a saliva test for these levels.

B. Estrogen Dominance with Progesterone Deficiency

If you scored high in this category, you likely have too much estrogen relative to your levels of progesterone. These two hormones, as dance partners, provide balance for one another. When estrogen tries to dance without its partner progesterone, the results are chaotic and hazardous.

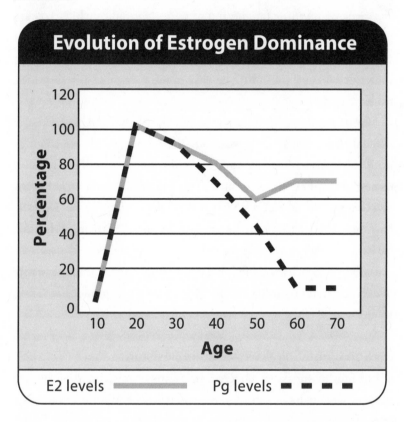

Beginning at about age 35, a woman's ovaries fail to produce sufficient progesterone. This is generally followed by a much slower decline in estrogen production, which leads to an imbalance or low progesterone-to-estrogen ratio. This imbalance, if untreated can cause a long list of symptoms, including the ones listed in section B of the pretest above, and can result in more serious disease such as breast and endometrial cancers, and bone loss. The good news is that this imbalance is easily corrected by supplementing with bioidentical hormones along with healthy lifestyle choices.

C. Adrenal Fatigue

As you might have guessed, scoring high in this category means you're fatigued. By the time you've reached this stage, you have likely been experiencing morning fatigue and weariness for quite awhile. You are probably sick and tired of being sick and tired. Due to prolonged stress of one kind or another, your adrenal glands are no longer producing sufficient cortisol, the hormone that is most essential for sustained healthy energy levels.

Similar to other endocrine glands like the thyroid and pancreas, the adrenal glands can actually wear out. The adrenal glands can adapt to meet the demands of high stress for years, but eventually after long-term duress, you will lose ground. This condition is often overlooked by conventional medicine and treated as depression. Those who suffer from adrenal fatigue are likely good friends with their local coffee baristas. Though a complete recovery from adrenal fatigue depends on a number of decaffeinated factors, supplementing with small amounts of cortisol along with healthy lifestyle choices can produce amazing results.

D. High Blood Sugar with Insulin Resistance

While insulin imbalance can creep up on you, women often experience sudden, unexplained, substantial weight gain in the hips and waist once the imbalance reaches a critical level. Unfortunately, this fat accumulation leads to a need for more insulin, something that is already in short supply when you have this condition. The fat cells around our midsection are the most insulin resistant fat cells in our body, meaning the pancreas must produce more than normal amounts of insulin to maintain an optimal blood sugar level.

While normal levels of insulin secretion create a healthy metabolic state in the body, excess insulin secretion leads to tissue breakdown, high blood pressure, and heart disease. If this situation is not reversed, the pancreas will eventually fail, blood sugar levels will rise out of control, and adult onset diabetes will develop bringing with it associated chronic diseases like kidney, eye, and heart disease. Reversing this process can be a challenge, but it is most achievable with hormone supplementation, nutritional adjustments, and exercise. You *can* reverse the momentum of this condition.

E. Low Metabolism and Subclinical Hypothyroidism

Scoring high in this category means you have a slow, inefficient metabolism connected with low thyroid function. Fatigue due to low thyroid function occurs most often toward evening, and is accompanied by many of the symptoms listed in the pretest. Even though you may have been told your blood tests for thyroid hormone levels are normal, actual function of the gland may still be suboptimal, or below where it needs to be. Thyroid gland function is one of the most misunderstood systems by conventional medical doctors. Regaining full thyroid function requires a willingness to strive for *optimal* hormone levels rather than *normal* levels. Minimal thyroid hormone replacement can go a long way to improving energy levels and well-being. For more information on thyroid function, see "What About Iodine Deficiency, Estrogen Dominance, and Thyroid Function?" on page 46.

F. Testosterone Deficiency

Too little testosterone doesn't just cause a lack of sexual desire, it may also deplete a woman's energy, vitality, and bone mineral content, leading to osteoporosis. Because testosterone is considered a male hormone, this deficiency is often overlooked in women, but optimal testosterone levels are crucial for women as well as men. With the right supplementation, you can once again feel young and vital.

G. Human Growth Hormone Deficiency

While human growth hormone (HGH) deficiency isn't normally associated with perimenopausal or menopausal symptoms, it relates in its potential for increasing longevity and quality of life. As well, it is an effective treatment for osteoporosis, a condition prevalent in menopausal women. Human growth hormone is an important piece in understanding the puzzle of aging and disease. At age 35, HGH declines exponentially in both women and men, stabilizing at age 60. When HGH is deficient, all of the other hormone pathways and organ functions are adversely affected.[67] Every bodily function tested, including the endocrine system, has been shown to benefit from optimal hormone levels. After all, recall the vitality you had at age 20 compared to age 50, and by age 70 it is that much worse. The decline in HGH is primarily responsible for the aging process.

There is currently a strong movement to challenge the aging process by supplementing with HGH. Unfortunately, however, the only proven effective method of sustained benefit is through daily subcutaneous injections and this is cost prohibitive for most people.

For those who can afford the injections, there are three bioidentical options. One includes the exact number of amino acids (191) made by the pituitary gland and a second is one amino acid short (190). Both are genetically engineered and free from infectious disease risk.[68] A third option is becoming more available. It increases growth hormone production in the brain. Its generic name is sermorelin. This is a hormone analog of Growth Hormone Releasing Hormone (GHRH), which is produced in the hypothalamus and stimulates the pituitary gland to produce more HGH. There are advantages to sermorelin, because it more closely mimics our natural physiology.[69] Unfortunately, like bioidentical HGH, sermorelin is expensive and requires daily injections. Nevertheless, all humans would likely benefit from more youthful levels of HGH at any age beyond 35. While expensive, boosting growth hormone represents an intriguing new frontier in turning back the body's biological clock.

Now that you have done some self-assessment about whether you are experiencing hormone imbalance and specifically which of your hormones may be out of balance, it is time to learn about the process of getting tested, finding a practitioner that can guide you through the process, and what lifestyle action steps will best support your particular hormone imbalance.

◄ **4** ►
Getting Support and Getting Tested

I f you are serious about your hormone health and scored within the 6–21 range on the pretest in the previous chapter, "What Are Your Hormones Doing," you will want to find support for adjusting your hormone levels and getting tested. If you don't see a physician that already does saliva testing and bioidentical hormone replacement therapy (BHRT), finding one in your community is your first step.

This may be your greatest challenge. However, we will discuss possible long distant options. Because the saliva tests are done in your own home and mailed to the lab, and pharmacies can mail prescriptions, it is possible to work with a physician or other trained healthcare provider by phone after an initial in-person visit. Whether in person or long-distance by phone, you will need to maintain an ongoing relationship for follow-up support to adjust your prescriptions as needed.

Because bioidentical hormone balancing is relatively new and practiced almost exclusively by physicians committed to natural medicine, your current primary care physician or gynecologist may not know about BHRT or saliva testing for measuring hormones. If this is the case, you have two avenues to pursue, educating your current doctor, or finding one who is already trained. If you have a strong relationship with your doctor and would like to work with him or her on this aspect of your health, we suggest you share this book with your doctor. There is a physicians' guide at the end of the book that provides all the information your doctor will need to become familiar with BHRT and saliva testing.

If, however, your doctor isn't trained or comfortable prescribing BHRT, you can find the resources you need to proceed, regardless of where you live. You may just need to be a little more resourceful in locating them. You may even be surprised to find other medical doctors, naturopathic physicians, physician's assistants, nurse practitioners, or pharmacists in your area who work with bioidentical hormones. Or there may be other health professionals—chiropractors, nutritionists, acupuncturists, and personal trainers who can help direct you to someone. There are plenty of resources out there, and with the resources provided in this book you should have little trouble making the connections you need to get started.

Find a Physician or Health Care Practitioner Who Prescribes Bioidentical Hormones

Ideally, you will be able to locate a physician in your community who is already working with bioidentical hormones. He or she will be able to order the necessary tests, tailor a prescription of hormones to correct your imbalance, and periodically monitor your hormone levels to keep you on track. (Remember, your hormone picture is continually evolving.) Be sure that whomever you end up working with understands your goals and is committed to using bioidentical hormones, not manufactured hormones (e.g., Premarin, Provera, or the two combined PremPro).

To determine if your current physician can help you, ask him or her to conduct a saliva test. Don't be frustrated if your physician isn't familiar with saliva testing. Unfortunately, many conventional physicians aren't familiar with saliva testing and therefore don't use it. As with many facets of medicine, inertia to change can be an obstacle to getting the most effective healthcare available. Medical schools continue to teach young doctors to use blood tests even though saliva testing was recognized back in the early 1980s as a more effective means for measuring hormone levels.

If your doctor is open to learning more in order to help you, ask him or her to read this book. Chapter 7 is written specifically for physicians as a guide for hormone testing and prescribing bioidentical hormone replacement therapy.

Finding BHRT-Trained Practitioners

If there is no one testing hormone levels and prescribing in your area, or you don't know how to go about finding someone, there are several avenues to explore.

The American College for Advancement in Medicine (ACAM)
www.acam.org

ACAM is a fellowship of complementary and alternative practitioners. The ACAM website has a search function to locate providers by city, state, distance from a zip code, and name. Areas of interest or specialties are included in the list of practitioners.

The American Association of Naturopathic Physicians (AANP)
www.naturopathic.org/findannd.php

Its find-a-physician function will help you find naturopathic physicians by city, state, zip code, or last name. You can then click a doctor's name that comes up in the search and find out about his or her location, type of practice, and areas of emphasis, including BHRT.

The International Academy of Compounding Pharmacists (IACP)

http://www.iacprx.org/site/PageServer?pagename=lookup_survey

A non-profit organization that protects compounding pharmacists from the pharmaceutical companies attempting to destroy compounding pharmacy as a profession. The IACP website has a function "For Patients" to locate a local compounding pharmacist. Some compounding pharmacists do limited BHRT consultations, or can refer you to a provider in your community.

John R. Lee, MD, Web Site

www.johnleemd.com/store/resource_finding.html

Dr. Lee's Web site offers resources for contacting BHRT doctors, compounding pharmacists, and a contact list of professional organizations that can guide you to finding a doctor.

Finding a Compounding Pharmacist in Your Area

If you can't find a local practitioner, look for a compounding pharmacy by checking the yellow pages under "pharmacies," or possibly "pharmacies—compounding." You can also check online by using those same keywords in your search engine. If you find a compounding pharmacist, they will be a good source for finding doctors or practitioners in your community that prescribe bioidentical hormones. If they know of no local practitioners, these pharmacists may be able to help you get tested and started on the basics—several hormone preparations are considered food (progesterone, DHEA) and are therefore not regulated and don't need a doctor's prescription. (For more information on compounding pharmacists, see "What is a Compounding Pharmacist" on page 37.)

Check Out Your Local Health Food Store

If you haven't already checked them out, your local health food store can be a great place to network on health issues and needs. It may even have a natural pharmacy department that carries bioidentical hormones or formulates bioidentical hormone prescriptions. Ask for the manager of the natural pharmacy or supplements department, look for a bulletin board that posts business cards of holistic practitioners, or ask for referrals and ideas for how to get tested and monitored.

Found a Doctor in the Know?
Now Get Tested

Once you have found a physician or practitioner who will support you in balancing your hormones, the next step is getting your hormone levels tested. What your hormone levels are doing on any given day of the month is different for every woman. Before you can restore the balance, you must first have an accurate picture of what your hormones are doing. The initial test will establish a baseline hormone profile, and two or three follow-up tests will give you the feedback needed to adjust your hormone levels until optimized. Before you know it, no more symptoms.

Why Saliva Testing: Saliva vs. Blood

The best way to measure hormone levels is through saliva. While hormones can be measured in blood and urine, neither of these mediums are as accurate for testing free, active hormone levels as saliva, which is precise, noninvasive, easy to do at home, and affordable. Also saliva testing is the only effective method for monitoring topical (absorbed through the skin by way of a cream or gel) hormone supplementation.

The greatest advantage of saliva testing is its ability to measure free, biologically-active hormone levels. Blood serum tests reflect total (bound) hormone levels, whereas saliva picks up that small percentage of hormone that is the active, or unbound, portion. It is this active portion that translates into information about hormone's functional levels rather than stored levels. A blood test will mainly tell you how much inactive hormone you have.

Blood testing for steroid hormones is so ingrained in allopathic training that converting MDs over to saliva may be like trying to move a mountain. The first article in the peer reviewed allopathic medical literature that clearly showed saliva testing for cortisol (a steroid hormone) to be preferred over blood was published in 1983, yet, we still encounter resistance to the concept, and this is despite even more current publications validating this concept.[70–72] Of course cortisol is only one of the steroid hormones accurately assessed in saliva and we use all five in our practice routinely.

There are a few blood tests that measure free active hormone levels, but they are expensive and technically difficult. Saliva, on the other hand, measures only free hormone. The salivary gland acts like a sieve and filters the blood carrier proteins out, letting us measure the free hormone directly. Most hormones are bound to protein and therefore are not accessible to the target organ, for example, the heart or brain. Knowing the free unbound levels is paramount to knowing if treatment is necessary and how much hormone to give to achieve balance.

Other Advantages of Saliva Testing

Saliva testing requires no needles, and you can collect the sample in the convenience of your own home, or anywhere. This is especially important for taking timed samples that require you to coordinate with a particular phase of the menstrual cycle, or for collecting multiple samples throughout the day.

Saliva testing also allows doctors to accurately monitor topically applied, cream or gel-based hormones, the preferred route of administration. Topically applied hormones act fast; they catch a ride on the red blood cells just under the skin and get transported and deposited directly into the body's organs, bypassing the liquid phase of blood (serum). In fact, they are measurable in saliva within 30 minutes.

Saliva testing involves pooling four samples taken at different times during the day, providing an average for estradiol, progesterone, testosterone, and DHEA levels. Because a woman with hormone imbalances typically experiences significant fluctuation during a single day, averaging makes for a far more accurate picture.

What Will the Test Measure?

A baseline saliva test measures life-sustaining steroid hormone levels. Included are estrogen (estradiol), progesterone, testosterone, DHEA, and morning cortisol. Depending on your history and symptoms, your doctor may also check your adrenal gland function by testing for noon, evening, and night cortisol levels. All of these hormone pathways are closely related and directly affect one another.

What to Expect: Taking the Saliva Test

The test kit generally comes in a box with four small snap-top plastic tubes, and a short questionnaire and instruction sheet. You collect a small amount of saliva in each of the plastic tubes at four prescribed times within a single day. This takes two to three minutes per tube. The test sometimes needs to be taken during a specific time of a woman's cycle. For menstruating women, it is best to test 4 to 6 days following ovulation, which translates to days 19, 20 or 21 of a 28-day cycle. The first day of your period is considered day one. The interval between days 19 through 21 typically represents the optimal time to measure estrogen and progesterone levels during ovulation—the period when progesterone production peaks. Progesterone levels are key to determining whether or not estrogen dominance is a problem. Baseline testosterone, DHEA, and cortisol levels can be tested any time during the menstrual cycle. Once a woman stops menstruating and enters menopause, she can test at anytime.

After all samples have been collected, they are placed in the provided shipping container and mailed to a certified lab. Results are then mailed directly to you and your doctor, usually within a week or so.

A Word of Caution

Make sure you or your doctor only use an accredited and CLIA-certified lab, one that uses FDA-approved saliva methods. There are many laboratories that use test systems designed for blood. These systems are not sufficiently sensitive to accurately read saliva concentrations. Some labs use methods that are home cooked and not subject to second-party scrutiny and approval. When performed correctly, saliva testing is the most accurate method for measuring all of the steroid hormones.

Formulating and Filling Your Prescription

With test results in hand, you are ready to have a bioidentical hormone formula tailored precisely to your needs. Once you get a prescription from your doctor, you will need to take it to a compounding pharmacy to be filled. The compounding pharmacists will then mix the precise amounts of each prescribed hormone into a single prescription.

While you can take hormones by pill, sublingually, or under the tongue in liquid form, or topically, we most often recommend using creams because they are convenient, well tolerated, and effective. Hormones absorbed through the skin bypass the liver. Otherwise, in oral preparations, a portion of them will be metabolized in the liver before ever reaching their desired location. Initially avoiding the liver makes absorption far more efficient.

Monitoring Levels and Adjusting Prescriptions

Once you begin taking your first prescription, you are in the home stretch, but not quite at the finish line. Because everyone absorbs hormones at different rates, you will need to have your hormone levels monitored and prescription adjusted as your hormone picture evolves. This will insure optimum results. With most patients, we find that one or two follow-up tests are sufficient to optimize hormone levels.

We recommend re-testing hormone levels after two months taking the initial prescription. As well, it is important to monitor any changes in symptoms to further determine if the prescription is still at the right level for optimal results. A follow-up test will establish that the target organs are receiving the appropriate amount of hormone, not too much or too little. We recommend retesting and reevaluating every two months until balance is achieved. This usually takes one to three visits with your practitioner.

What Should You Expect Taking Bioidentical Hormones

You should expect nothing less than to recover your youthful vigor with major, if not complete, resolution of the related symptoms you reported prior to starting bioidentical hormone replacement therapy. It is not uncommon for our patients to exclaim, "I have my life back!" or for spouses to call to say, "My partner is her old self again," or for spouses to make an appointment to get started on their own path toward hormone rebalancing.

◄ 5 ►
Off the Edge
Correcting the Problem

Now let's get you off that hormone imbalanced edge for good. Our goal is to not only help you correct your hormone imbalance with bioidentical hormones, but to suggest effective dietary, herbal, and lifestyle modifications for improving your overall health and well-being for the rest of your life. While we are committed to relieving your challenging mid-life symptoms, rebuilding and sustaining a strong foundation of health will assure greater outcomes when taking bioidentical hormone replacement therapy.

If you are like many of our patients, you may have already sought answers in conventional medicine and come up short. You may have been put on synthetic hormone replacement therapy (HRT), been told you were depressed and given an antidepressant, or worse yet, been told there is no treatment, and your symptoms would pass in time. While well intentioned, the current medical model for treating hormone imbalances leading up to and including menopause is often misguided and, in some cases, even dangerous. More importantly, it not only doesn't offer the symptom relief you so desperately seek, but also doesn't address underlying causes that accentuate perimenopausal and menopausal symptoms.

The good news is that bioidentical hormone replacement therapy (BHRT) is a safe and effective alternative to conventional HRT. But because it is not yet widely known and understood, using BHRT will require initiative and a determination to stay empowered in your efforts. You will need to be proactive and continue to educate yourself.

While we recommend that you work with a health care practitioner in your area, in person, you can find someone outside your area and work with them long distance. You can get all the support and guidance needed for the basics through phone consultations. Testing is done through the mail and you can receive results by e-mail or mail. If you need to go to a lab for blood tests, you can get those done through your primary care doctor and send copies of the results to the healthcare practitioner you are working with on hormone balance. Another option is to offer this book to your current primary care physician as a guide to providing you the help you are seeking. Chapter 7 is a physicians' reference guide covering everything your doctor needs to know to diagnose and treat your particular hormone imbalance.

What follows is a comprehensive guide to treating your hormone imbalances holistically using bioidentical hormones, while making strategic adjustments to your diet and lifestyle. The specific saliva and blood tests associated with each hormone imbalance is also listed. There is a resources and tools section for further research on each imbalance in Appendix A.

You can take dietary action steps immediately, before beginning bioidentical hormone treatment. With bioidentical hormone replacement therapy or not, the included recommendations can help you build and maintain long-term hormone health. We encourage you to find your imbalances below, explore them each in more detail, and begin to take action.

Building the Foundation for Hormone Health

There are five basic building blocks for good hormone health and, for that matter, health in general. Whatever your hormone imbalance, there are health promoting actions that will support and enhance the effectiveness of your particular treatment program.

1. Eat Well and At the Right Times

There is no one dietary protocol that fits every human being's nutritional needs, although working with patients over the past couple of decades, as well as staying current with the medical research, it is clear that any well-founded and sound dietary approach will have a few things in common. It will reduce or eliminate foods that cause inflammation in the body, and it will support glucose and insulin regulation.

Good, stable blood sugar levels are essential for stabilizing emotions and physiology, including hormone levels. There are two facets to this: eating the right foods and eating at the right times. Ironically, it is often more difficult to remember to eat well and thoughtfully during times of emotional turmoil created by fluctuating hormones. Nevertheless, if you practice healthy eating habits when you are not under the spell of erratic hormones, you will be more likely to remember those habits when they do take over.

Eating a wide variety of whole foods, representing all the colors of the rainbow, is a rule of thumb for healthy eating. In Japan, this premise is considered so essential that the government provides guidelines that spell out the minimum number of different foods one should consume daily for optimal health. For adults, fifteen different foods are recommended per day.[73]

Eating well also means avoiding processed foods that include additives and sugars that can wreak havoc on blood sugar and energy levels. Avoid refined white foods like baked goods made from white flour and white sugar; processed grains like white rice and pasta; and other refined and processed foods. Instead, choose brown, or whole grain rice, and whole grain wheat pastas and breads. If you crave sweets, eat fruit or use honey, fruit juice concentrate, or sucanat (dried cane juice) in place of white sugar when making desserts. Eating whole foods will slow the rate at which your body metabolizes them, providing for more even, constant energy levels. Rapidly rising and falling blood sugar levels directly relate to energy and mood swings.

When and how often we eat also affects our health. Our bodies love rhythm and consistency. It is best to eat a minimum of three meals a day spaced approximately four and a half hours apart. In addition, those of us who are more sensitive to blood sugar fluctuations need snacks between those three meals. By eating on a regular schedule, you prime your body's insulin pump (the hormone that helps you transform sugar into energy) to be constant and even.

2. Minimize Stress Where You Can

Slow down! We live in a culture that pressures us to do more and do it faster. We recommend you make a conscious effort to challenge that message. Make a discipline out of slowing down and being fully present for each moment of your day—especially when the cues are to speed up. Allow yourself to fully relax, for example, when sitting down to a meal or driving to the next activity. Program yourself to turn the on switch off whenever you can, even if for only a few minutes. Some people find that a 10-minute nap at lunch can make a world of difference in the quality of their day. Be creative about how you work this into your days, but make it a conscious goal. Your adrenal glands will thank you.

Practice breathing deeply. It's probably the last thing on your mind when you feel anxious or pressured to keep all balls in the air, but short shallow breathing actually feeds stress and anxiety. It's simple, no books to read or classes to take. Start by lying down on the floor on your back with your knees bent so that your belly remains soft. Close your eyes and rest. Your body will automatically take you into deeper belly-centered breathing, after a few moments of resting. Memorize this feeling. Notice how different this breath is from the unconscious breathing that comes when you are busy with your day, distracted by harried thoughts.

3. Drink More Water

Made up mostly of water, our bodies rely on a steady input to assure that our overall metabolism works smoothly and efficiently. Think of it as your physiologic lubricator. Also, there is no better source for your daily fluid needs. Your specific water needs vary depending on several things, your weight, how much you exercise each day, climate, temperature extremes, alcohol consumption, whether you are pregnant, or whether you are sick with a fever or diarrhea. Also, approximately 20 percent of our water comes from the food we eat, and if you eat a healthy diet, you can adjust water intake accordingly.

On an average, assuming no unusual or extreme conditions, you need to drink approximately 64 ounces, or 8 glasses, of water daily for optimal health. You can also calculate the amount of water you need by dividing your weight in half and converting that number to ounces. If you weigh 140 pounds, you would want to drink 70 oz. of water daily.

Remember, the quality of the water you drink is also important. If possible drink only filtered water, rather than from your tap. Although it can be challenging, avoid drinking from plastic containers, particularly the soft ones. Xenoestrogenic (estrogen-like) chemicals contained in plastics leach into the water.

It is important to divide up your daily water intake throughout the day. This is particularly important if you exercise heavily. If you have a kidney or adrenal problem, or you are taking diuretics for any reason, you need to consult with your physician about how much water to drink each day.

4. Exercise Regularly

Exercise, or simply move, enough to elevate your heart rate for 20 to 25 minutes three to five times a week. This alone will create positive physiological changes in your body, which in turn promotes hormone health. If you don't exercise your muscles, including your heart muscle, they atrophy; you loose them. The same is true of the glands that make our hormones. Exercise is vital to all our body systems.

If you can't work in a trip to the gym three times a week, look for other ways to move your body and raise your heart rate. Find a low maintenance alternative that fits into your daily routine. You could buy a pedometer to count your footsteps. If your office is on the 8th floor (or the 2nd floor for that matter), make a point of taking the stairs. Or instead of taking a coffee break, head out the door and walk briskly for 10 minutes. Find a lunch destination, near work or home, that is a 20-minute walk away, and make a point of walking to lunch several times a week. Set goals using your pedometer to motivate yourself to take more steps. Reward yourself for achieving each milestone goal.

5. Reduce Stimulants and Alcohol

Reduce or stop using coffee, soda pop, chocolate, tea, and alcohol. Even if you are fatigued from hormone fluctuations, caffeine provides only a brief boost, and it is a costly temporary gain. The net effect, fatigue and anxiety, are actually worsened over the long term. Alcohol stresses the liver, which is then less able to process hormones such as estrogen, making balance maintenance that much more difficult. Also as a refined form of sugar, alcohol adversely affects blood sugar and insulin levels, both key factors in hormone balance.

Coming Back to Balance:
Causes, Remedies, and Action Steps

Here in lies the pearl of your discovery. Once you understand the cause of your imbalance, you can remedy it. The following information provides you with the specific remedies and action steps you need to take to regain hormone balance, as well as your overall health.

We recommend that you share this book and its recommendations with your caregiver whether they are familiar with bioidentical hormone replacement therapy or not. If they are not familiar with BHRT make sure they peruse "Chapter 7: Physicians' Reference Guide: Understanding Salivary Testing and Bioidentical Hormone Treatment Protocols."

For best results, it is important to use saliva testing for steroid hormone (estrogen, progesterone, testosterone) levels. Saliva is by nature essentially free of interfering proteins; free or unbound levels are readily tested. Serum (blood) testing, conversely, includes interfering proteins that bind hormones, skewing values by including bound and unbound level values. (*See* "Chapter 4: Getting Support and Getting Tested.") Saliva collection is stress-free (no needles) and can be taken at home at a particular time of the month or several times throughout the day, as needed.

Anti-Inflammatory Diet:
A Dietary Building Block for Re-balancing Your Hormones

Below is an outline for a basic anti-inflammatory diet, which serves as the foundation for correcting all the hormone imbalance conditions. As you begin to incorporate these foods and remove others, there are a couple of simple issues of food quality to remember. Select fresh foods whenever you can. If possible, choose organically grown fruits and vegetables to eliminate pesticides and chemical residue consumption. Rinse fruits and vegetables thoroughly.

If you select animal sources of protein, look for free-range or organically raised chicken, turkey, or lamb. Trim visible fat and prepare by broiling, baking, stewing, grilling, or stir-frying. Cold-water fish, like salmon, mackerel, and halibut, is another excellent source of protein and omega-3 essential fatty acids; important nutrients in this diet. If you do not tolerate fish, talk to your healthcare practitioner about possible substitutions. He or she may suggest supplemental fish oil. Avoid shellfish, as they may cause allergic reactions.

Anti-inflammatory Diet

Foods to Include	Foods to Exclude
Fruits: unsweetened fresh, frozen, or water-packed canned fruits, fruit juices (except those specifically prohibited)	All citrus fruits: oranges, grapefruits, lemons, limes, grapes, fruit drinks, dried fruit
Starches: non-gluten grains, brown rice, millet, quinoa, amaranth, teff, tapioca, buckwheat	Wheat, corn, oats, barley, spelt, kamut, rye, and all gluten-containing products
Breads and Cereals: any made from rice, buckwheat, millet, soy, tapioca, arrowroot, amaranth, quinoa	All wheat, oat, spelt, kamut, rye, barley, or gluten-containing products

Meats: all fresh fish such as halibut, salmon, cod, sole, trout; wild game; chicken; turkey; lamb	Beef, pork, cold cuts, frankfurters, sausage, canned meats, eggs, shellfish
Legumes: all dried beans, peas, lentils	
Nuts and Seeds: almonds, cashews, walnuts, pecans, sesame seeds, sunflower seeds, pumpkin seeds, flaxseeds, whole or as nut and seed butters	Peanuts, peanut butter, pistachios
Dairy Products: milk substitutes such as rice milk, soy milk, nut milk	Milk, cheese, cottage cheese, cream, yogurt, butter, ice cream, frozen yogurt, non-dairy creamers
Vegetables: raw, steamed, sautéed, juiced, or baked vegetables (except those specifically prohibited)	Canned, or creamed in casseroles; nightshade family vegetables including tomatoes; all potatoes (except yams or sweet potatoes); eggplant; red, green, or yellow bell peppers
Fats: olive oil, flaxseed oil, coconut oil, safflower oil, sunflower oil, sesame oil, walnut oil, pumpkin oil, almond oil, and dressings made from these oils	Margarine, butter, shortening, processed oils, hydrogenated oils, salad dressings, mayonnaise, spreads, canola oil
Beverages: 8 cups of filtered or distilled water per day, herbal tea	Soda pop, alcoholic beverages, coffee, tea, all caffeinated beverages
Spices: cinnamon, cumin, dill, garlic, ginger, oregano, parsley, rosemary, tarragon, thyme, turmeric	Cayenne pepper, paprika

Sweeteners: brown rice syrup, fruit sweetener, molasses, stevia	No white, brown or refined sugar, honey, maple syrup, corn syrup, and especially high fructose corn syrup

Hidden sources of food allergens:
- Cornstarch in baking powder and processed foods
- Corn syrup solids or maltodextrin (or derivatives) used as sweetener
- Grain vinegar in ketchup and mustard
- Oats or corn in amaranth and millet flake cereals

Shopping List—Anti-inflammatory Food Choices

Proteins

chicken, lamb, turkey, fish (cod, halibut, mackerel, salmon, trout, tuna, wild game), legumes (dried beans, dried peas, lentils), soy (soy milk, soy yogurt-casein free, tofu, tempeh)

Grains

amaranth, millet, quinoa, rice, rice bread, rice cakes, rice cereals, rice milk, rice pancakes, rice pasta, tapioca, teff

Vegetables

alfalfa sprouts, artichokes, asparagus, avocados, beets, bok choy, broccoli, brussels sprouts, cabbage, carrots, cauliflower, celery, chard, cucumber, daikon radish, endive, escarole, green or yellow beans, green-mustard, jicama, kale, kohlrabi, leeks, lettuce, mung beans, okra, onions, parsnips, radishes, rutabaga, sea weed (kelp), snow peas, spinach, squash (summer, winter), sweet potatoes, taro, turnips, water chestnuts, yams, zucchini squash

Fruits

apple, applesauce, apricot, avocado, banana, blueberries, cherries, kiwi, mango, melon, nectarine, papaya, peach, pear, pineapple, plum, prune, raspberries, strawberries

Sweeteners

brown rice syrup, fruit sweetener, molasses, stevia

Nuts, Seeds, and Oils

almond oil, almonds, coconut oil, cashews, flax oil, hazelnuts, olive oil, pecans, pumpkin oil, pumpkin seeds, safflower oil, sesame oil, sunflower oil, sunflower seeds, walnut oil, walnuts, butters of these nuts and seeds

Spices

anise, bay leaf, basil, cardamom, celery seed, cinnamon, cumin, dill, dry mustard, fennel, garlic, ginger, marjoram, oregano, parsley, rosemary, saffron, savory, tarragon, thyme, turmeric

Now that you have the ingredients for a generally healthy and hormone-balancing diet, read on to find specific dietary and laboratory test action steps for each specific hormone imbalance. Included are condition-specific lists of beneficial foods and foods to avoid. Many of you will find yourselves dealing with more than one condition related to hormonal imbalance. If this is true for you, add the lists together, being sure not to eat foods listed under any of the avoid lists.

If you have a question about a particular food, check to see if it is on the food list. Do not make substitutions except those outlined in these instructions or recommended by your practitioner. You should, of course, avoid any foods to which you are intolerant or allergic, even if they are listed in this diet. (For more in-depth information on the anti-inflammatory diet, refer to Dr. Jessica K. Black's book, *The Anti-Inflammation Diet and Recipe Book*.)

Estrogen Deficiency

Lisa, 49

> *For two months Lisa had been waking each night at about 2:00 a.m., her heart pounding and forehead damp with sweat. During the day she felt extremely tired and anxious. She often found herself obsessing about details or things people said (even to the point of paranoia). We tested her hormone levels and prescribed bioidentical hormones in a topical cream. She also began a moderate exercise program (3x per week for 30 minutes) and started eating more whole foods. Six weeks later, she described the difference in her quality of life as, "night and day. I feel like myself again!"*

The Cause

Estrogen deficiency is not as common as one might think. Estrogen deficiency is a problem for only about 20 percent of women entering menopause, and it is even less likely that estrogen is the only hormone imbalance. What more commonly occurs in women with low estrogen are simultaneously low levels of other hormones such as progesterone and testosterone.

Symptoms of low estrogen include hot flashes, night sweats, and vaginal dryness. Estrogen deficiency can also cause fatigue, memory problems, and foggy thinking—but these same symptoms can also be caused

by estrogen dominance (too much estrogen). Because the bladder is sensitive to estrogen, a deficiency may also make bladder and urinary tract
problems worse. Some women also report uncontrollable tearing or
runny eyes, which is due to lachrymal (tear duct) sac shrinkage.

The bottom line is that our bodies clearly function best with an optimum level of estrogen. In addition to all of the functions it serves to
support a woman's reproductive ability, estrogen aids memory. Studies
on Alzheimer's disease and estrogen have shown that estrogen has the
capacity to create an excitatory effect on the brain, enhancing mental
activity.

Estrogen affects brain activity in a number of ways. Acute exposure
to estrogen in juvenile rat brains shows a marked increase in metabolic
activity, potentiating neuronal activity.[74] Also, the cerebral blood vessels of rats respond to estrogen by producing nitric oxide (NO), which
leads to vasodilation and increased blood flow. The relative loss of NO
production is thought to play a role in the development of dementia including Alzheimer's Disease.[75] When a woman in menopause is
chronically stimulated by estrogen that is inadequately unopposed by
the calming effects of progesterone, it is understandable why she may
be on edge, or irritable as many women describe it.

The Remedy

The first step to achieving optimum estrogen balance is to get your hormone levels tested. We recommend using saliva testing for all sex hormones, which is discussed in detail, along with information on finding
a trained healthcare provider or educating your doctor, in the previous
chapter "Getting Support, Getting Tested."

It is ironic that in an era of widespread hormone replacement therapy, women are not only put on estrogen before being tested, they most
often receive a standard dose. One size does not fit all. The amount you

need may vary widely depending on your particular hormone fluctuations, which are based on age, body weight, nutrition, and other factors.

If your estrogen levels turn out to be low, a trained practitioner can prescribe bioidentical estrogen. There are several widely available bioidentical products on the market, including Bi-Est, a combination of two bioidentical estrogens, estriol and estradiol. In addition to relieving symptoms, bioidentical estrogen supplements will help keep your bones and cardiovascular system healthy. These supplements come in two forms, topical preparation or pharmaceutical patches. They are easy to use and often provide immediate, dramatic results. Rebalancing your body's estrogen will have many beneficial effects, including quieting hot flashes and night sweats, shoring up a weepy disposition, and enhancing your sense of well-being.

Note: if there is a history of breast cancer in your family history, we advise you take a more conservative approach to supplementing with estrogen, even with bioidentical estrogen, because increasing estrogen levels can increase your risk of breast cancer.[76]

Action Steps
Whole Foods as Medicine
Proteins

- fish
  - bonito
  - eel
  - flounder
  - halibut
  - salmon
- legumes
  - great northern beans
  - kidney beans
  - navy beans

- lentils
  - black
  - red
  - yellow
- soy
  - miso
  - soy nuts
  - tempeh

Grains

- arrowroot
- brown rice
- buckwheat
- flaxseeds
- oats
- popcorn
- rye

Fats

- black currant oil
- evening primrose oil
- fish oil
- flaxseed oil
- pumpkin seeds

Vegetables

- beet greens
- broccoli
- cabbage
- chard
- collard greens
- eggplant
- green beans
- hominy
- mustard greens
- pumpkin
- romaine lettuce
- spinach
- tomatoes
- winter squash

Fruits

- apples
- apricots
- cherries
- dates
- honeydew melon
- kiwi
- mango
- papaya
- pineapple
- pomegranate
- prunes
- raspberries

AVOID

- alcohol
- animal fats
- caffeine
- dairy products
- hydrogenated oils
- spicy hot foods

Salivary Hormone Panel

- cortisol (a.m., p.m.)
- DHEA
- estradiol
- estriol
- progesterone
- testosterone

Blood Tests

- CBC
- lipid panel: VAP
- metabolic chemistry panel
- thyroid: TSH, fT3, fT4 (f = free)

Other Resources

See "Appendix A: Resources and Tools: Stacking the Deck."

Estrogen Dominance with Progesterone Deficiency

Betty, 47

A registered nurse, Betty came to us gripped by perimenopausal symptoms. Over the previous year and a half, she had been experiencing hot flashes, night sweats, irregular periods with heavy bleeding, sadness and irritability, breast enlargement and tenderness, mental fog, and increased forgetfulness. She headed into work one morning and found herself standing in the supermarket without knowing why she was there. This so alarmed her that she made an appointment with us for help. Fortunately, she had heard about the conventional hormone replacement therapy (HRT) study that had been cancelled due to dangerous side effects and chose to seek an alternative.

We tested her saliva for estrogen and progesterone, among other hormones, and discovered she was experiencing estrogen dominance. Her estrogen level was more than adequate, but there was insufficient progesterone to balance it. Prescribing a topically applied cream of progesterone and monitoring her hormone levels through saliva testing readily corrected the problem. Within two months, all of her symptoms were reduced by 90 percent. That was five years ago and now we only see Betty once a year to recheck her hormone levels and refill her prescription.

The Cause

The symptoms caused by too much estrogen, or estrogen dominance, are too often mistaken for low estrogen. Not having your hormone levels tested can lead to misdiagnoses by untrained, or ignorant medical doctors. Taking additional estrogen, of course, only makes matters worse in this case.

Estrogen dominance is the most common hormone imbalance as you near menopause. The ovaries undergo clear hormonal changes as you progress through the menstrual years, and the balance between the two hormones that regulate its function—progesterone and estrogen—shifts. Beginning at age 35, progesterone and estrogen levels drop gradually as ovarian function declines. Progesterone plummets precipitously at menopause when the ovaries essentially stop functioning altogether. Eventually, you stop producing progesterone altogether, with the exception of a small amount secreted by the adrenal glands. If you want to retain the positive benefits of progesterone, you must, at some point, take it as a supplement.

The balance between estrogen and progesterone can be further compromised as women age, because the production of estrogen switches from the ovaries to fatty tissue where testosterone is converted into estrogen, further exacerbating the potential for high estrogen levels. Being overweight as you enter perimenopause and menopause makes you that much more susceptible to estrogen dominance.

The Remedy

The first step to correcting the problem is to get your hormone levels tested. This establishes a baseline indicating your current hormone status, and will serve to point your doctor toward what is needed to bring you back to an optimal progesterone/estrogen ratio. We recommend using saliva testing for all five steroid hormones, which is discussed in detail along with information on finding a trained healthcare provider or educating your doctor in the previous chapter "Getting Support, Getting Tested."

The remedy for fixing your imbalance is simple, supplement your body's progesterone level. Bioidentical progesterone is readily available, safe, and effective, and easily taken as a topical cream or gel. It is derived from plant hormones (phytohormones) and is identical in structure to the progesterone made by the ovaries. Because it is not assimilated well through the intestinal tract, progesterone is best applied directly to the skin where it is readily absorbed and delivered to the organs that need it: breasts, uterus, vaginal mucosa, and brain. Progesterone opposes the effects of estrogen, which is why it is important for protecting the uterus from the cancer-causing effects of too much estrogen. The goal of progesterone replacement is to achieve a balance between estrogen and progesterone.

In addition to taking progesterone, you can also create a healthier hormone balance by following the action steps outlined below. The suggested foods will minimize estrogen-containing foods in your diet. Also, see "What About Iodine Deficiency, Estrogen Dominance, and Thyroid Function?" on page 46.

Action Steps
Whole Foods as Medicine

Proteins
- fish
  - halibut
  - salmon
  - sardines
  - shrimp
  - tuna
  - yellowtail
- legumes
  - black beans
  - garbanzo beans
  - kidney beans
  - navy beans
  - pinto beans
- soy
  - edamame
  - miso
  - soy nuts
  - tempeh
- texturized vegetable protein

Grains
- amaranth
- arrowroot (kudzu)
- brown rice
- bulgar
- corn tortillas
- flaxseeds
- quinoa
- rye

Fats
- olive oil
- fish or cod liver oil
- flaxseed oil

Vegetables

- algae
- asparagus
- bok choy
- brussels sprouts
- cauliflower
- celery
- cucumbers
- kale
- lettuce
- mushrooms
- okra
- onions
- snow peas
- sweet potatoes
- zucchini

Fruits

- cantaloupe
- cranberries
- guava
- nectarines
- pears
- plums
- raspberries
- starfruit
- strawberries
- watermelon

AVOID

- alcohol
- beef
- caffeine
- chicken

- dairy
- refined sugar
- spicy hot foods

Salivary Hormone Tests

- cortisol (a.m., p.m.)
- DHEA
- estradiol
- progesterone
- testosterone

Fasting Blood Tests

- CBC
- lipid panel: VAP
- metabolic chemistry panel
- thyroid: TSH, fT3, fT4 (f = free)

Urine Test (24-hour challenge)

Iodine spot and load
(If you suspect an iodine deficiency connection, or also suffer from low thyroid function.)

Other Resources

See "Appendix A: Resources and Tools: Stacking the Deck."

Adrenal Fatigue

Bella, 43

Bella started to wonder if she was depressed. She was tired even as she woke up in the morning. She forced herself through each workday only to return home to plop down on the couch. She felt too tired to fix dinner or even change out of her work clothes. She watched TV, ate fast food, and fell asleep on the couch. On a scale of one to ten, she reported her energy level as a three. Prior to the last year, she would have characterized herself as a high-energy person.

Her periods became irregular and heavy. She started experiencing cyclical headaches three days prior to her period, lasting up to a week after her period began. We tested her saliva for hormone levels to assess her sex and adrenal hormones.

Based on results we prescribed an adrenal protocol along with a bioidentical hormone cream containing progesterone and DHEA. Within three weeks, she reported that her energy had risen from a three to a six on a scale of one to ten. As her adrenal glands healed, she felt more solid. Again, her interest in socializing and pursuing creative hobbies returned.

The Cause

Excessive stress has a profound impact on hormonal cycles and your adrenal glands. Those little organs that sit on top of your kidneys take the brunt of stress. Our primitive survival glands, the adrenals, provide the energy that feeds our fight or flight response when faced with danger. Hundreds of years ago, the danger might have been a real physical threat, such as becoming prey to a hungry tiger. Even though most of us no longer have to defend our lives on a daily basis, our physiology still reads certain levels of stress as life threatening. When overly stressed, we can get stuck in a perpetual fight or flight state, eventually depleting our adrenal vitality. This, in turn, leads to hormone imbalance and a host of symptoms: fatigue, irritability, anxiety, and frequent illness—this is before factoring in the hormonal imbalances of menopause, which exacerbate these symptoms.

Demands in our lives have increased substantially from even a generation ago. One hundred years ago our great grandmother's adrenal tests would likely have been dramatically different from our own. While their lives undoubtedly involved hardship, our great-grandmothers probably had more physiological stability because the pace of life was slower and their environment didn't shift as much. Today we experience alarm in rush-hour traffic, ringing cell phones, and the hyper-drive speed of information exchange. Even at home we absorb images of terrorism and violence on the nightly news. In each of these situations, our bodies mount a chemical readiness to respond to stress. But, because these are false alarms as life and death alarms go, the stress is never resolved. We never truly relax after or between alarm responses. Eventually one leads into the next, and before we realize the pattern, we're stuck in high gear, a chronic condition that eventually wears out our adrenal reserves. Once the reserve is gone, our bodies produce significantly less cortisol and DHEA, both of which regulate our energy levels.

Adrenal fatigue has far-reaching implications. Not only is fatigue a consequence, but premenstrual syndrome (PMS) and postmenopausal symptoms are worsened. Working with women in our practice, we often find that until adrenal gland function is corrected, balancing sex hormones (estrogen, progesterone, and testosterone) and relieving symptoms of their imbalance is often impossible.

The Remedy

The first step to correcting the problem is to get your hormone levels tested. This will help establish a baseline for where your levels are now and point you toward what is needed to bring them back into an optimal ratio. We recommend using saliva testing for all sex hormones and cortisol levels. Testing is discussed in detail along with information on finding a trained healthcare provider or educating your doctor in the previous chapter "Getting Support, Getting Tested."

Because adrenal glands are regulated by a primitive part of the brain, rejuvenation may take longer than other more superficial body systems. Sometimes termed the waking-day hormone, cortisol regulates a vast array of systems and functions in the body, including blood sugar levels and inflammation. They are an important building block for health and well-being. Convincing the body to produce an optimal level of cortisol—the hormone secreted by the adrenals—once depleted can be tricky, but it is possible. These are resilient glands designed to adapt and recalibrate to meet life's fluctuating demands.

We can sometimes solve the problem by providing nutrient support to the adrenals. To function well, for example, Vitamins C, B5, and B6 are necessary. Depending on the severity and other existing health problems, simply adding these supplements and adjusting your diet, may improve your symptoms. These supplements provide the adrenal glands with the precursors they need to make cortisol. The adrenal glands often can rebound with this level of support if nutrient replacement occurs before the glands scar from overstress.

If nutritious support doesn't work, taking small amounts of cortisol as a temporary measure can sometimes increase adrenal function. This is physiologic rather than pharmacological dosing, something we call priming the pump. The goal is to stimulate the adrenal glands to pick up the pace, rather then take over their job. The brain has to make a decision about whether it will produce more cortisol, and small amounts of cortisol can actually stimulate the adrenal glands to make more cortisol. But we have to be careful during this process, because if we give the body too much cortisol it gets lazy and stops producing cortisol itself altogether. This is the very thing that occurs when patients take synthetic cortisone, like prednisone, for extended periods of time.

Once compromised, adrenal glands can take anywhere from six months to two years to rebuild. That said, you might begin seeing positive changes within as little as three weeks after beginning a program to restore normal function. However, if adrenal scarring is extensive, you may need to take cortisol indefinitely. Even if that is the case, there is no need to despair. It is like taking a thyroid hormone replacement when the thyroid gland begins to fail. Because we live much longer than we did a century ago, you can expect some organ systems to fail as you age. As with all hormone replacement therapies, choosing bioidentical hormones is safer and more effective, as they are fully recognized by our bodies as biologically compatible.

Action Steps
Whole Foods as Medicine

Proteins
- eggs
- fish
- fowl
- legumes
- meat

Fats
- flaxseed oil
- olive oil
- safflower oil
- sunflower oil

Vegetables
- beet greens
- celery
- green beans
- kelp
- onions
- peppers, hot red
- spinach
- swiss chard
- tomatoes
- zucchini

Grains
- amaranth
- barley (unpearled)
- brown rice
- buckwheat
- millet (unhulled)
- oats (whole)
- quinoa
- whole wheat

Fruits
- apples
- cherries
- grapes
- kiwi
- mango
- papaya
- pears
- plums

Nuts and Seeds (raw only)
- almonds
- flaxseeds
- hazelnuts
- pumpkin seeds
- sesame seeds
- sunflower seeds
- walnuts

AVOID
- alcohol
- caffeine (all stimulants)
- nicotine
- processed luncheon meats
- refined carbohydrates (low glycemic index foods)

Salivary Hormone Tests
- cortisol (a.m., noon, evening, p.m.)
- DHEA
- estradiol
- progesterone
- testosterone

Fasting Blood Tests
- CBC
- metabolic chemistry panel
- thyroid: TSH, fT3, fT4 (f = free)

Other Resources
See "Appendix A: Resources and Tools: Stacking the Deck."

High Blood Sugar and Insulin Resistance

Daisy, 13

As a young teen, Daisy began her day with two bowls of sugary cereal or three chocolate-glazed donuts. She drank two 2-liter bottles of cola every couple of days along with cartons of chocolate milk. She binged on candy and potato chips while hiding under the bed. She ate an average of four fast food meals each week. She stood 4'8" tall and weighed 130 pounds.

Her mother, Maria, called her a little round ball. Daisy's blood glucose level often topped 400 mg/dl (normal fasting blood glucose is <110 mg/dl and diabetes is diagnosed at 126 mg/dl or above). Even though she was still a child, Daisy was diagnosed with Type 2 diabetes—a condition formerly known as adult-onset diabetes.

The Cause

Insulin helps the body use glucose (sugar) from the blood. Insulin can be likened to the key that unlocks the door (receptor) to the cell, allowing glucose to pass into it from the blood. Once inside the cell, glucose is either used for energy or stored for future use in the liver and muscle cells (glycogen). Insulin resistance occurs when the normal amount of insulin secreted by the pancreas is no longer enough to open the doors to the cells. It is not known why this happens, but once it does the body secretes even more insulin to try to maintain normal blood glucose levels (hyperinsulinism). Insulin resistance symptoms begin to occur due to the increase in circulating glucose and insulin.

High blood sugar is brought on by genetics, a diet of refined sugar, and hormone imbalance. Some of us are born with a biochemistry that doesn't metabolize sugars well. When this is combined with over-consumption of refined sugars and the hormone shifts that come with menopause, the body produces too much insulin. This, in turn, leads to a condition where the body actually resists its own hormone (insulin) for absorbing sugars, causing weight gain (belly fat) and a host of other symptoms.

The pancreas makes insulin, a hormone that moves sugar from the blood into our cells. Without insulin, sugar builds up in the blood—which is essentially the condition known as insulin resistance. The pancreas interprets this condition as a need for more insulin, so it releases more insulin. The increased production of insulin is able to compensate for the imbalance of sugar for a while, but the pancreas, as other endocrine glands such as the thyroid and adrenals, will eventually fail from overuse. The pancreas has a finite capacity to produce insulin. If triggered to over-produce insulin as a result of too much sugar in the diet, the pancreas' functional capacity will eventually become exhausted. It may quit producing insulin all together, resulting in diabetes. Excess insulin also leads to high blood pressure, which contributes to heart and kidney disease.

Some people are born with a condition known as sugar sensitivity. These people are likely to come from families with a high incidence of alcoholism, depression, and/or diabetes—all signs of a metabolism that does not absorb sugars well. Their metabolisms set them up for a love/hate relationship with sugar and make them vulnerable to developing insulin resistance.

Pre-diabetes, insulin resistance, and metabolic syndrome are common medical terms used for this predisposition. In women, this condition may lead to fatigue, weight gain (particularly around the middle of the body), mood swings, headaches, sugar cravings and binges, low libido, and excess androgen (testosterone and DHEA) production, which causes increased facial/body hair, acne, and scalp hair loss. Not all people with insulin resistance develop diabetes. By maintaining a healthy weight and a physically active lifestyle, adult-onset diabetes is far less likely.

Though falling progesterone is a key factor in developing insulin resistance, testosterone imbalance and increased cortisol levels (stress-related condition affecting the adrenal glands) can also be significant contributors. Optimal testosterone levels are essential: they aid insulin (made in the pancreas) in pushing glucose out of the blood stream and into our cells.

The Remedy

You can reverse the outcome of insulin resistance through hormone balancing and a commitment to diet and lifestyle changes. There is a transition period between having a functioning pancreas and developing diabetes, during which you can reverse the disease course and regain pancreatic function. By taking action now, you can prevent diabetes, lose weight, and feel better than ever.

The first step to correcting the problem is to get your hormone levels tested. This will help establish a baseline status of your current levels and point you in the direction needed to regain an optimal ratio. We recommend using saliva testing for all five steroid hormones, which is discussed in detail along with information on finding a trained healthcare provider or educating your doctor in the previous chapter "Getting Support, Getting Tested."

The key to reversing the effects of insulin resistance is to reverse the collection of fat around the middle of your body. This will require fat loss everywhere, but most importantly the insulin resistant fat around your mid section. This will, in turn, reduce your body's need for insulin. Losing this weight is complex. Progesterone in standard dosages will help reduce fat collection around the middle of your body, but the physiology is complicated by changes in fat metabolism that occur with falling hormone levels, specifically progesterone.

Progesterone can be thought of as a braking system for the collection of fat around the thighs and abdomen. So when these levels fall, fat in form of free fatty acids collects in the fat cells around the belly and hips. For women deficient in progesterone, which is a majority of perimenopausal women, supplementing with bioidentical progesterone helps restore balance and correct negative fat metabolism.

You can generate the greatest positive impact on insulin levels by making dietary changes. A plant-based, whole food, low-fat diet with no refined (white) sugar will make a world of difference.[77] A combination of dietary discretion, exercise, and bioidentical hormone supplementation will help you lower body weight drastically and correct the trend toward diabetes.

That exercising muscle needs less insulin is an added incentive for making a commitment to regular exercise. Muscle can use insulin to convert sugar into energy, while fat resists insulin and requires more of it to convert that same sugar. The more muscle mass you have and the more you work them, the less insulin is required from the pancreas to maintain blood sugar levels.

To get a full picture of where you are in the continuum of insulin resistance, you need to take both blood and saliva tests. The blood tests will measure fasting blood sugar (glucose), insulin, and lipids (fatty components). The saliva test will measure testosterone and DHEA levels.

Action Steps
Whole Foods as Medicine
Proteins

- chicken (hormone-free)
  fish (cold water)
  cod
  halibut
  mackerel
  salmon
  tuna
  trout
- lamb (hormone-free)

- legumes
  dried beans
  lentils
  peas
- soy
  miso
  tempeh
  tofu
- turkey (hormone-free)

Grains

- basmati rice
- brown rice
- millet (unhulled)

- oats
- quinoa
- rye

Vegetables (non-starchy)

- bok choy   *Limit to 2x week*
- broccoli   - carrots
- cabbage   - peas
- cauliflower   - sweet potatoes
- celery   - squash
- daikon radish   - yams
- endive
- escarole
- jicama
- kale
- lettuce (all green leafy vegetables)

Fats

- olive oil
- cod-liver oil
- flaxseed oil
- grape-seed oil

Fruits (2x week)

- apples (tart only, e.g., granny smith, pippins)
- blueberries
- pears (firm, e.g., bosc, d'anjou)

Nuts (raw only)

- almonds
- hazelnuts
- walnuts

Sweetners

- brown rice syrup (sparingly)
- molasses (sparingly)
- stevia

AVOID

- beef
- cane sugar
- canned meats
- cold cuts
- corn syrup (high fructose)
- dairy products (especially cow's milk)
- dried fruit
- frankfurters
- fruit drinks
- fructose
- pork
- sausage
- soda pop

Salivary Hormone Tests
- cortisol (a.m., noon, evening, p.m.)
- DHEA
- estradiol
- progesterone
- testosterone

Fasting Blood Tests
- CBC
- metabolic chemistry panel
- insulin
- lipid panel: VAP
- thyroid: TSH, fT3, fT4 (f = free)

Other Resources
See "Appendix A: Resources and Tools: Stacking the Deck."

Low Metabolism and Hypothyroidism

Martha, 54

> *Martha complained for months of continuously feeling cold, experiencing evening fatigue, weight gain, constipation, brittle hair and nails, markedly reduced libido, and hair loss. Once postmenopausal, her primary care provider tested Martha's thyroid levels and claimed they were normal. She was offered an antidepressant, which she refused. During our examination, we observed many signs of low thyroid gland function (low temperature, scalloped tongue, dry skin, thick brittle hair, and sluggish reflexes). In addition to thyroid-stimulating hormone (TSH), we tested her levels of free T3 and T4, which indicated that her thyroid levels were*

actually below normal. Because our medical practice focuses on optimizing health, we prescribed a combination of thyroid hormones in a low dose and adjusted it over a three-month period until vitality returned and symptoms resolved. As well, her hot flashes and night sweats completely resolved. Correcting thyroid function enhances the effectiveness of bioidentical hormone replacement.

The Cause

Many women suffer from the effects of a sluggish or ineffective thyroid system, but there is more to the problem. Thyroid hormones' effect on the rate of metabolism within the cell is profound and relies on sufficient levels of progesterone, estrogen, and cortisol. For cell doors to open, a four-pronged hormone key is required. Thyroid, estrogen, progesterone and cortisol are all needed to turn a cell on. As we have said, progesterone production falls with age, beginning most notably around age 35, and essentially stops at menopause. Based on the four-pronged key requirement, symptoms that are typical of thyroid deficiency can sometimes by corrected by taking progesterone. Similarly, cortisol is required for normal thyroid function. For the thyroid hormone to work its magic on individual cells, cortisol must be at sufficient levels. Cortisol is made by the adrenal glands, which are often over taxed due to stress. Though estrogen deficiency is less common, when present, supplementation is important as well.

There is another peculiarity with the thyroid hormone system. The thyroid gland primarily makes and releases the hormone T4, which is the inactive thyroid hormone. The most active hormone is T3, which the liver makes by converting T4 to T3. Think of T3 as the business end of the thyroid—it makes the deal that converts the hormone into a form that the body can most readily use. Because this transaction occurs in the liver, its health becomes an important player in optimal thyroid function as well. An inflamed or toxic liver can reduce T3 production, and because conventional lab tests don't include measuring T3 values, this problem is often not identified.

Conventional methods of testing for slow metabolism or hypothyroid condition miss detecting this problem in at least 25 percent of the population. If you are one of these individuals, you may have repeatedly been told that your thyroid gland was normal because the result of your standard blood test, testing only TSH, was within the normal range. That only indicates that the thyroid gland itself is producing enough thyroid hormone (T4). What the test does not reflect is the status of the liver to convert T4 into active thyroid hormone (T3). This conversion happens at a cellular level and our best screening for this value is to measure basal body temperatures and muscle reflexes. Low thyroid leads to retarded muscle reflexes everywhere—most conveniently tested at the knee or behind the foot. These physical findings coupled with the clinical history and adrenal function panel results can help a skilled practitioner diagnose and treat either underproduction of thyroid hormone or poor conversion of T4 to T3.

The Remedy

To understand the nature of your low metabolism and hypothyroidism, you'll need blood, urine, and saliva tests. The blood tests should include thyroid-stimulating hormone (TSH), thyroid peroxidase (TPO) antibodies, free T3 (most active thyroid hormone), and free T4 (least active thyroid hormone). Unlike other hormones, thyroid testing must be done with blood serum (the straw-colored liquid phase of blood). The urine test is a 24-hour iodine loading evaluation. Saliva testing is also helpful because symptoms of low metabolism can be mimicked or aggravated by estrogen dominance and hypoadrenia, or under active adrenal glands.[78] Estrogen, progesterone, DHEA, and cortisol level testing are also recommended.

Be aware that most conventionally trained practitioners are not trained in the subtleties involved in suboptimal thyroid gland function and the interactions among T3, T4, progesterone, and cortisol. Nor are they generally aware of the prevalence of iodine deficiency. Screen your provider carefully if you suspect hypothyroid is an issue. With conventional thyroid testing you could have a TSH level of 5.4 (most lab's normal reference range is 0.4 to 5.5) along with every known thyroid hormone deficiency symptom and still be told you are not thyroid hormone deficient. The reality is that the higher the TSH level, the more likely your body is deficient in either or both T4 and T3. It is important that you find a practitioner with a deeper understanding of hypothyroidism and the importance of addressing functional imbalances and hormonal optimization.

Typically, when we find low or suboptimal T3 levels and replace them with bioidentical T3, women experience renewed energy and vitality. A combination of T3 and T4 (thyroid hormone) supplement can help correct an ineffective or sluggish metabolism. Once again, be aware that thyroid hormone supplementation, even in the natural or holistic medical community, is often misdirected by limiting therapy to T4 replacement only. It has been our experience that a combination of T4 and T3 preparation tailored to the individual is far more effective, while remaining as safe.

Remember in any hormonal imbalance, healthy diet and lifestyle choices play critical roles in achieving optimal results. In particular, with low thyroid function, iodine supplementation may be warranted. See "What About Iodine Deficiency, Estrogen Dominance, and Thyroid Function?" on page 46 for information on the importance of sufficient iodine levels in our diet.

Action Steps
Whole Foods as Medicine
Proteins
- fish
  - bonito
  - halibut
  - mackerel
  - salmon
  - sole
  - tuna

- soy
  - miso (white)
  - soybeans (raw)
  - tofu (extra firm)

Grains
- barley
- buckwheat (kasha)
- kamut
- oats
- quinoa

Fruits
- apples
- apricots
- cranberries
- grapes
- strawberries

Vegetables
- bitter melon
- cabbage
- carrots
- carrot tops
- dried kelp (konbu)
- seaweed (nori)
- sweet potato (purple)

AVOID
- brominated foods (source: fumigated grain and its
  products, commercial baked goods)
- chlorinated water

Salivary Hormone Tests
- cortisol (a.m., noon, evening, p.m.)
- DHEA
- estradiol
- progesterone
- testosterone

Fasting Blood Tests
- lipid panel: VAP
- metabolic chemistry panel
- thyroid: TSH, fT4, fT3, TPO (f = free)

Urine Test (24-hour challenge)
Iodine spot and load

(If you suspect an iodine deficiency connection, or also suffer from low thyroid function. For more information see "What About Iodine Deficiency, Estrogen Dominance, and Thyroid Function?" on page 46.)

Other Resources
See "Appendix A: Resources and Tools: Stacking the Deck."

Testosterone Deficiency

Susan, 53

> *Susan was wondering what she could do to increase her sex drive, which had dropped to about 25 percent of what it had been. She went from enjoying, initiating, and engaging sexual activity with her husband up to four times a week to having no interest in sex and only becoming active because she felt guilty about meeting her husband's needs (once every couple of weeks). Susan used to work out at the gym five days a week, but over the past year, she had nearly stopped going to the gym because she felt tired and weak. We tested her sex hormone*

saliva levels and found she was deficient in both progesterone and testosterone. We prescribed a bioidentical transdermal cream, and one month later Susan reported feeling strong and confident again. Her sex drive was much better, back to about 75 percent of what it used to be, and she returned to working out at the gym three days a week.

The Cause

Women who come to us to address change-of-life symptoms often chuckle about their record low sex drive level. Not because it's funny, but because they recognize it as a stereotypical symptom of menopause. The waning interest in sex clearly has chemical ties to reproduction and ovulation. As those cycles begin to wind down and testosterone levels fall, sex drive wanes. Women with low testosterone may also have a diminished interest in their appearance, and may find that wrinkling is occurring at an accelerated rate. They may also discover they have poor hair texture, decreased bone mass, decreased energy, increased cellulite, and increased anxiety. Even though testosterone is usually thought of as a male hormone, deficient levels can also compromise a woman's ability to achieve optimal health. Despite the fact that women have only about one-eighth of the testosterone that men have, maintaining the right level of testosterone is essential for stamina, muscle strength, bone density, and libido.

The ovaries and adrenal glands are the primary sources of testosterone in women, sharing production equally. The luteinizing hormone (LH) that initiates ovulation also stimulates cells surrounding and in between the developing follicles to produce testosterone. In addition to making testosterone, these cells have a supportive structural function; they provide the ground substance, or stroma, for the ovaries.

Without the foundation these cells provide, the ovaries would collapse. These stroma cells become less responsive to hormone stimulation as a woman ages. They shrink, eventually losing their ability to function. As this process evolves, the testosterone produced by the ovaries drastically declines, causing lost libido, vaginal dryness, and decreased bone density and muscle tone.

Interestingly, as the LH rises and progesterone production falls during the transition to menopause, there is a temporary increase in testosterone. The brain keeps trying to produce an egg (elevated LH) even though the ovaries are preparing to close up shop. This explains the increase in facial hair, acne, and scalp hair loss that many women experience during perimenopause. Sustained elevations of testosterone can also occur with insulin resistance, also known as metabolic syndrome.

The Remedy

Once you have determined the precise testosterone level through saliva testing, testosterone supplementation can quickly enhance your sex drive, confidence, stamina, and sense of well-being. Don't worry, supplementing testosterone, or a precursor like DHEA, does not mean you will grow a beard and start fist fights in the parking lot. With the right physiological dosing, you'll simply return to an optimum level of function for your body, without side effects.

DHEA, sold over-the-counter is the hormone women most readily convert to testosterone. One way to increase testosterone levels is to supplement with DHEA. However, the body can also convert DHEA into estrogen, making it important to work with a trained healthcare practitioner. You need to get tested and monitored to determine the best course for your particular situation.

The first step is to determine your DHEA and testosterone levels through saliva testing. We recommend using saliva testing for all five steroid hormones, which is discussed in detail along with information on finding a trained healthcare provider or educating your doctor, in the previous chapter "Getting Support, Getting Tested."

Action Steps
Whole Foods as Medicine

Proteins
- fish
  - cod
  - salmon
  - sardines
  - sea bass
  - tuna
- fowl and game
  (organic, grass-fed)

- goat milk and dairy
  products (organic)
  - milk
  - yogurt
- legumes
  - lima beans
  - split peas
  - white beans

Grains
- amaranth
- brown rice
- buckwheat
- millet
- quinoa

Fats
- almond oil
- grape-seed oil
- peanut oil
- sesame oil
- walnut oil

Vegetables
- artichokes (not Jerusalem)
- asparagus
- beets
- broccoli
- brussels sprouts
- cabbage
- carrots
- cauliflower

- eggplant
- garlic
- onions
- peas
- peppers
- pumpkin
- squash

Fruits
- apples
- bananas
- blueberries

AVOID
- beef
- corn
- cow's milk
- hormone-injected chicken and turkey
- potatoes

Salivary Hormone Tests
- cortisol (a.m., p.m.)
- DHEA
- estradiol
- progesterone
- testosterone

Fasting Blood Tests
- CBC
- insulin
- metabolic chemistry panel
- SHBG

Other Resources
See "Appendix A: Resources and Tools: Stacking the Deck."

Human Growth Hormone Deficiency

Jennifer, 42

Jennifer had experienced debilitating fatigue and muscle pain for more than a decade. She sought medical care through the usual channels seeing five different practitioners and specialists. She was diagnosed with fibromyalgia and prescribed standard synthetic medicines such as antidepressants. Needless to say, she was very frustrated by the time she walked through our door. After a thorough medical evaluation, we determined she was deficient in human growth hormone (HGH). We searched the medical literature and found convincing evidence that supplementing with human growth hormone would be worth trying. At Jen's eight-week follow-up visit after receiving the optimum growth hormone dosage, she had regained essentially 100 percent of her function. She declared emphatically, "I have my life back." That was five years ago and she continues to report excellent health.

The Cause

It seems that our biological clock is often out of sync with our desire to stay healthy and vital beyond its wind-down point. What good is a retirement plan if the master plan is for us to get ill and die just about the time we retire? The clock is programmed, some might say unfairly, to wind down too early, leaving us vulnerable to chronic debilitating disease or cancer. The software program in our brain, the hypothalamus, directs the aging process through the decreased production of growth hormone, the master hormone.

Growth hormone levels peak at age 20, begin to fall at age 30, and decline approximately 14 percent a decade thereafter, leveling off at age 60. If you are 35 years or older, you have likely observed the startling effects of this decline on your beauty and stamina. There is no telling how long human beings could live if our growth hormone stayed at a 20-year-old's level. If our bodies were to have all the nutrients required to thrive—including growth hormone—we might live to ages of biblical proportions.

The Remedy

Presently the best remedy for aging is a daily injection of human growth hormone (HGH). The first step is to assess your HGH production. This helps establish a baseline value and the correct dosage for HGH supplementation. A word of caution: testing your HGH production can be challenging, because HGH fluctuates drastically throughout the day, making a single test result subject to error. However, nature has helped us out with insulin-like growth factor 1 (IGF-1), which is the biologic mediator of HGH. IGF-1 levels only fluctuate eight percent throughout the day. A single serum test measuring IGF-1 is an effective approximation of overall growth hormone production and will help monitor replacement therapy.

Genetically engineered, infectious disease-free HGH can help turn back the biological clock. However, there is a drawback. HGH is expensive and it has to be injected daily. Be skeptical of Internet-based claims of HGH products that can be applied to the skin, swallowed, sprayed up your nose, or administered under the tongue. These products provide, at best, a transient benefit. It is only a matter of weeks before the benefit of these forms of HGH, if there is any, will wear off completely.

Short of injecting growth hormone, there are other ways to stay young. Longevity is, to a great degree, controlled by exercise and nutritional habits. Exercise is critical to healthy hormone levels, including HGH. It is important to stay active and exercise regularly. Good nutrition is another factor. For example, patients with malnutrition due to anorexia nervosa have an abnormal response to the growth hormone they produce and greatly benefit from recombinant growth hormone administration.[79] Dr. T. Colin Campbell and associates, in their sentinel book, *The China Study*, clearly demonstrates the benefits of a plant-based, whole food, low fat diet on longevity. Such a diet reduces the risk of cancer, heart disease, diabetes, and autoimmune disease. (*See* "Chapter 6: Redefining the Aging Process: Claiming 40 as the New 30" for a more in-depth discussion.)

Action Steps
Salivary Hormone Tests
- cortisol (a.m., noon, evening, p.m.)
- DHEA
- estradiol
- progesterone
- testosterone

Fasting Blood Tests
- CBC
- IGF-1, IGF-BP3
- metabolic chemistry panel
- lipid panel: VAP
- thyroid: TSH, fT3, fT4 (f = free)

Other Resources
See "Appendix A: Resources and Tools: Stacking the Deck."

◄ 6 ►
Redefining the Aging Process
Claiming 40 as the New 30

The current medical model is failing us. America spends more money per capita on health care than any country on this planet. Yet, the United States only ranks forty-first in life expectancy compared to other countries.[80] The saddest statistic is that we have the highest level of neonatal and infant mortality.[81] And that's not all. The U.S. medical system is the third leading cause of death in our country. There are 225,000 deaths per year attributed to iatrogenic causes (illness due to medical examination or treatment), ranking only below cancer and heart disease.[82] Of these deaths, 113,000 are caused by medicine errors in hospitals and adverse effects of medications, 7,000 and 106,000 events respectfully.[83]

No wonder most of the aging population is looking for longevity and quality of life without the risk of dangerous drugs. The movement is toward natural bioidentical therapies, supplementing the declining hormone levels that betray our youth and help lead us down the path to chronic illnesses. With saliva testing and bioidentical hormone replacement therapy, we currently have the tools to manage many of the negative effects of aging, including prevention of many chronic debilitating diseases.

If you are currently in perimenopause or menopause, you were most likely born between 1946 and 1967, which puts you in the baby boomer generation. There are 76.9 million Americans in this group who turn 50 at a rate of one every seven seconds, or 11,000 per day. By 2020, 40 percent of the U.S. population will be over the age 60. This generation is a sort of human tsunami hitting the current medical system. Overall, the baby boomers are not happy with our disease-oriented medical system. They are educated, physically active, and have the financial resources to demand a health system that focuses on prevention. Recall that the baby boomers have changed every institution that got in its way—Vietnam War, segregation, women's rights . . .

The current system would collapse if it were not for chronic debilitating illnesses such as diabetes, heart disease, and cancer. Hospitals' financial survival depends upon treating patients in the late stages of these illnesses. These diseases are, for the most part, preventable. Prevention is, quite frankly, not in the best financial interest of the pharmaceutical and hospital industries. The conventional medical model's attention is on illness, not wellness.

There is good news, however. A huge movement among health care practitioners, mostly outside of the conventional circles, is focused on wellness and is positioning itself to lead in a national, if not global, health care reformation. There are tens of thousands of natural, holistic, and medically trained providers throughout the United States and Canada who are highly motivated to help you find a better way to get well and stay well. (*See* "Appendix A: Resources and Tools: Stacking the Deck.")

Turn Back The Clock

What is old? It's likely that your current idea of aging is outdated. Your potential life expectancy is much greater than your parents'. Through hormone balancing, good nutrition, and exercise it is possible to extend your life by decades. You should be planning to live with vitality into at least your tenth decade. Instead of a rocking chair retirement, you may be considering another career, new hobbies, travel, or other experiences beyond your wildest dreams for life after 65. With the burgeoning new understandings of how to manipulate the aging process, the aging population can enjoy a more youthful level of energy, to live robustly, and continue to contribute to society at unprecedented levels.

Aging is a purposeful process. We might even think of it as a "disease" process that can be manipulated by hormones. The therapies discussed in this book may just be a starting point for you, once you regain your health. In addition to balancing waning and fluctuating sex hormones (progesterone, estrogen, testosterone), adrenal hormones (cortisol), and the blood-stabilizing hormone, insulin, discussed in these pages, you may also want to consider human growth hormone (HGH). HGH has been shown to effectively turn back our biological clock. While HGH is available at a high cost and must be injected to be effective, we expect a more patient-friendly delivery system developed in the near future. In the meantime, don't be taken in by the myriad of products offered on the Internet and by nutritional suppliers and health food stores. Injection is presently the only effective HGH delivery system.

Even while you look for the next breakthrough in hormone balancing, rest assured that following the simple steps outlined in this book will not only help prevent possible disease, but also help you make extraordinary strides toward enhancing your quality of life and longevity. Increasing quality of life and longevity is indeed a new frontier to explore and—with some help from bioidentical hormones—you will have the vitality to explore it!

◄ **7** ►

Physicians' Reference Guide
Understanding Salivary Testing and
Bioidentical Hormone Treatment Protocols

Whether you are new to the concepts in this book or are a trained and experienced natural or holistic physician, we wish you the very best. We hope that our paths cross somewhere in the future and that this book contributes to the success of your practice.

Our journey has been a rewarding experience of applying basic physiology to the understanding of chronic disease. We often tell our patients that their condition is not due to a deficiency of the antidepressant or synthetic hormone they have been prescribed. At the beginning of each new visit, we make it clear that we rarely prescribe any contrived chemicals to correct what we believe is an alteration of one's physiology. We do offer advice about correcting and rebalancing the body, to return it to a healthy state. This often includes supplementing hormones, which can return physiological function at levels that many patients had not imagined possible and a result they did not experience from the myriad of pharmaceuticals given to them by well meaning, but misguided physicians.

As the medical doctor in this partnership, I was one of those misdirected physicians for many years. My medical school training, received at one of the nation's most prestigious schools, University of California at San Francisco, basically taught me to identify symptoms and associate a pharmaceutical drug to correct it, prescribe it, and end the visit. There was essentially no holistic or preventive medicine training and not a word about bioidentical hormones as an option for treating perimenopausal and menopausal complaints. The last 10 years have taught me that my medical training, unlike Dr. Lommen's naturopathic medical training, limited my ability to safely and effectively help patients. Broadening my understanding of medical practice to include holistic and preventive health care has been the most rewarding shift as a doctor. A patient's whole being, listening to them, has become my focus; I no longer simply treat the laboratory results or prescribe pharmaceuticals.

Before covering the essentials of testing for hormone imbalances and protocols for treating with bioidentical hormones, we need to establish some common ground by defining terms.

Estrone (E1)

Metabolites of E1 are carcinogenic. E1 is in equilibrium with estradiol (E2) and therefore can be approximated by knowing the E2 level. There is virtually no need to ever supplement with E1.

Estradiol (E2)

The strongest form of estrogen; and when elevated, the form which is linked to breast and endometrial cancer. When deficient, supplementing it will readily modify symptoms of menopause, such as hot flashes, night sweats, insomnia, and emotional lability. It is best supplemented topically because PO supplementation is known to reduce the effectiveness of growth hormone.

Estriol (E3)

E3 is considered the weakest estrogen, but also the breast protective estrogen. It is used widely to treat vaginal dryness and atrophy, and as a safe estrogen replacement for breast cancer survivors. It is generally added whenever E2 is supplemented in the form of Bi-Est (usually 4:1; E3:E2). It is also considered neuro-protective for female multiple sclerosis patients.[84]

Estrogen dominance

A term popularized by John Lee, MD, to describe estrogen excess relative to progesterone (*see* Pg/E2 ratio below). It is now understood that estrogen dominance can occur at any stage in a woman's menstrual life, and virtually always occurs during PMS and menopause. (*See* E2 above for ill effects of excess E2.) Estrogen dominance is also recognized in males as a cause of prostate gland pathology. Also, see "What About Iodine Deficiency, Estrogen Dominance, and Thyroid Function" on page 46 to understand this often overlooked connection.

Progesterone/Estrogen Ratio

Estrogen dominance is most often diagnosed by measuring the saliva levels of Pg and E2 and then dividing Pg by E2. The resulting optimal therapeutic range of Pg/E2 is 200 to 600.

Progesterone (Pg)

The bio-identical hormone known to block the proliferative effects of E2, consequently helping protect breast and endometrial tissue. When replaced at physiological levels, it stabilizes mood, increases bone mineralization, reduces PMS and postmenopausal symptoms, and decreases the risk for breast and endometrial cancer.

Progestin or Progestagins

Progestins are proprietary synthetic progesterone analogs (e.g., medroxyprogesterone acetate) often referred to as part of HRT, which research has shown to cause dangerous side effects. They are associated with increased risk of breast cancer, endometrial cancer, heart attacks, strokes, liver tumors, blood clotting, and pulmonary embolism.[85] Patient compliance is extremely low with these analogs.

DHEA

Dehydroepiandrosterone is a steroid hormone secreted by the adrenal cortex and converts or stimulates the production of estrogens and testosterone.

DHEA-S

The circulating inactive polar precursor of DHEA. Because of its polarity it cannot be accurately assessed in saliva. There is no therapeutic value in testing for DHEA-S.

Androstenedione

A natural steroid hormone that acts as a precursor to testosterone and other androgens.

Testosterone

A female sex hormone produced in the adrenal glands and ovaries in significantly lower amounts then males, but with no less overall importance to maintaining healthy hormone balance.

Cortisol

A hormone produced within the adrenal gland's cortex created and released in response to stress or physical trauma modifying several diverse physiological responses including blood sugar levels, blood pressure, and heart rate. It also controls inflammation and modulates the immune response. Excess cortisol suppresses the immune system.

Saliva Testing for Hormone Levels

Since the theme of this book is primarily steroid hormone imbalances, consequences, and how to correct them, it is first important to clarify any misunderstanding about the accuracy and efficacy of saliva as a laboratory test medium. As a board certified pathologist, I can attest to the validity and accuracy of this test method when performed correctly. In fact, saliva testing is far superior to serum for diagnosing and monitoring treatment of steroid hormone imbalances.

The greatest advantage to using saliva for testing hormone levels is its ability to measure free, biologically active hormones. The majority of all hormones, particularly lipid (steroid) hormones, found in the blood stream are bound to proteins or stuck on the surface of red blood cells (RBCs). Because blood is essentially a water medium not easily mixed with fatty substances, these hormones must attach to a lipid-friendly protein or red cell membrane to be transported from the organ that produced it to its target site.

The total (bound) hormone levels measured in blood serum cannot reflect the hormones functional or active levels, causing inaccuracy in the tested hormone's actual physiological impact. Saliva tests, conversely, measure the small percentage of active, unbound hormone. There are a few blood tests that measure free hormone levels, but they are very expensive and technically difficult to do. A saliva test, on the other hand, measures only free hormone levels without any modifications. The salivary gland acts like a sieve and filters the blood carrier proteins and RBCs out, allowing us to measure the free hormone directly.

Saliva testing is simple. There are no needles required and it can

be done by a patient in the convenience of their own homes—or anywhere for that matter. This is especially important for taking timed
samples. Timing can be critical when measuring hormone levels that
fluctuate throughout a month or day, as do estrogen and progesterone
during the menstrual cycle, and cortisol during a 24-hour period.

Another major advantage of saliva testing is its compatibility for
monitoring topical, transvaginal, or sublingual hormones—the preferred route of bioidentical hormone administration. Topically applied
hormones act fast; they catch a ride on the red blood cells just under
the skin and get directly deposited in the body's organs.[62] In fact, they
are measurable in saliva within 30 minutes.

Also, after cortisol levels are determined, the four saliva samples
taken throughout a day can be pooled giving averaged values for estradiol, progesterone, testosterone and DHEA. Because of the unpredictable daily hormone fluctuations in a hormonally imbalanced woman,
this pooled sample gives a far more accurate reflection of hormonal
status.

Don't Overlook the Adrenal Connection: Cortisol, DHEA, and Adrenal Fatigue

It may be important to assess adrenal status (cortisol and DHEA) along
with sex hormones even when the chief complaints seem mainly to re-
side in sex hormone imbalance. The sex hormone pathways are closely
related to cortisol and DHEA and will directly affect one another.

Cortisol has a well-established 24-hour diurnal rhythm. The time
of day it is measured will reveal unique aspects of the patient's health.
If there are sleep disruptions, a p.m. cortisol test should also be performed, and if there are metabolic and blood sugar regulation problems
suspected, four test times will be useful: a.m., noon, evening, and p.m.

Although adrenal fatigue may not be on your list of possible diagnoses, consider the usefulness of testing for and treating low adrenal

function in patients with subclinical symptoms. The philosophy at my medical school, and perhaps yours, was pretty cut and dried. You either had "normal" adrenal function or you had Addison's disease. Also, I was taught to be fearful of glucocorticoid supplementation, which was justified, considering prednisone and other synthetics are very dangerous. However, the safe and effective supplementation of physiological doses of bioidentical cortisol was never discussed.

In my experience as a clinical pathologist, having reviewed tens of thousands of salivary adrenal function tests—DHEA and cortisol (a.m., noon, evening, p.m.)—and treating hundreds of patients, approximately 70 percent of these tests have shown some degree of insufficient cortisol or DHEA production or both.

When it comes to correcting chronic fatigue and pain, there is nothing more effective than supplementing hypoadrenic patients with physiological doses of cortisol. Many patients tagged with convenient diagnoses such as chronic fatigue syndrome and fibromyalgia often recover fully when given cortisol support. Our approach to adrenal insufficiency does not differ from our approach to thyroid hormone deficiency or diabetes, supplement appropriately with bioidentical hormones, promote a healthy whole foods diet, exercise, and stress management.

Saliva tests measured at four times throughout the day will show the circadian pattern of cortisol production. You should supplement with cortisol only when there is low cortisol. A person's symptoms can be made worse if they take a supplement and don't need it. The same caution should be noted with DHEA, which is an over-the-counter hormone. If it is not needed, we recommend it not be given. The body can convert DHEA into testosterone and estradiol; it is imperative to be intentional in treating the adrenal glands.

Also take caution, hypoadrenia and hypothyroidism share many of the same signs and symptoms and can be difficult to distinguish. This problem is compounded when both conditions exist, which is not uncommon, and the unsuspecting provider treats the hypothyroidism only to find that the therapeutic benefit is only transient. In fact, this may lead to a major energy crash if the hypoadrenia is not concomitantly treated. I highly recommend Dr. Jeffrie's and Dr. Wilson's books for further discussion. (*See* "Appendix A: Resources and Tools: Stacking the Deck.")

How It Is Done

To do saliva testing, the patient simply collects saliva into a small plastic tube at four prescribed times in a single day. Each collection takes two to three minutes. The test needs to be done during a particular time of a woman's cycle. For women who are menstruating, it is best to test 4 to 6 days following ovulation, which translates to days 19 through 21 of a 28-day cycle. If the cycles are regular, but either shorter or longer than 28 days advise the patient to provide the samples seven days before the expected onset of her period. Once all of the samples have been collected, they are placed in a shipping container and mailed to a certified lab. Results are available online, can be faxed, or mailed to you directly.

Which Hormones Should I Test?

Five-Hormone Panel

- estrogen
- progesterone
- testosterone
- DHEA
- cortisol (a.m.)

We believe the bare minimum for assessing hormonal status and endocrine function is the five-hormone panel, which includes estrogen, progesterone, testosterone, DHEA, and cortisol—a.m. When there are any sleep disruptions or high cancer risk profiles, we also recommend testing p.m. cortisol. But in general, as a basic guideline, an excellent starting place is the five-hormone panel.

As clinicians with over twenty-five years of experience working with natural hormone balancing and bioidentical hormone replacement therapy the reasons for this panel choice are well established and the intricate balance and direct relationship between adrenal gland function and sex hormone balance have proven out clinically. Frequently when estrogen, progesterone, and testosterone are showing deficiencies and excesses, the adrenal glands have already been working overtime in an attempt to compensate for reproductive system strain, as well as for other functional roles.

Initiating and maintaining waking day activity and function, a.m. cortisol levels represent the maximum output for the entire 24-hour period. DHEA has equally important duties and is often referred to as the anti-aging hormone because it is central in its role for disease prevention and health optimization. Measuring DHEA and a.m. cortisol is your first glimpse into the status of endocrine balance and function. As we age and our production of sex hormones changes, the adrenal glands maintain a central role in sustaining optimal health and function. Aging is often first noticed as sexual function diminishes and menopause begins. While it is obvious that we want to test estrogen, progesterone, and testosterone levels at this stage, it is not so apparent but equally important to also measure the two foundational hormones responsible for endocrine balance, cortisol and DHEA.

Although it is not a hormone, it also may be relevant to do a 24-hour urine-loading test for iodine deficiency when you have a patient with hormone imbalances consistent with estrogen dominance or hypothyroidism. A standard dose of iodine and iodide is ingested and the amount passed in the urine over 24-hours determines sufficiency. If a patient passes less than 90 percent of the loading dose he or she is deficient and would benefit from iodine and iodide supplementation. See "What About Iodine Deficiency, Estrogen Dominance, and Thyroid Function" on page 46 to further understand this often-overlooked connection.

Bioidentical Hormone Replacement

Once you know what imbalances you are dealing with, the next decision is to choose a route of administration. Bioidentical hormone replacement therapy means individualized prescriptions, combinations, and forms of hormones created to fit the particular needs of each patient. There is no one-size-fits-all as there is in conventional HRT prescription. With options available, you can tailor, or compound, a formula for your patient and choose the most effective route.

Routes of Administration

Oral

When swallowed, sex hormones (estrogens, progesterone, and testosterone) are either poorly absorbed by the gastrointestinal tract or are metabolized and consequently deactivated by the liver before they can exert their biological effect. In fact, synthetic or pharmaceutical hormones are often toxic to the liver for that very reason, for example, methyltestosterone. Fortunately, bioidentical hormones are effectively absorbed through the skin, oral cavity, or vagina. On the other hand, cortisol and DHEA are effective taken orally and frequently are administered that way.

Often overlooked, estradiol, even the bioidentical form, when given orally lowers insulin-like growth factor one (IGF-1). Since IGF-1 is the biologic mediator of human growth hormone HGH, this is a very unfavorable side effect. As we were educating ourselves about the use of HGH in our practice, we serendipitously discovered 10 references in the peer reviewed medical literature to support the occurrence of this side effect.[86] For this reason, we rarely use oral estradiol, preferring topical or transdermal therapy. Note: A portion of sublingual hormone preparations is swallowed.

Intervaginal

Vaginal application, though effective, is often not as convenient for patients as the other routes of administration. The vaginal formulas are limited to suppositories or creams, both of which are often unsatisfactory to women.

Nasal

Nasal application, though a theoretical option, is not practical when considering the volume of the preparations needed and the challenge to manage the resultant nasal discharge.

Injection

Injections, aside from being painful, are limited essentially to testosterone, which, for women, can instead be prescribed in a topical application.

Topical

Topical application is by far the most popular route for hormone supplementation. There are three primary reasons:

1. Bioidentical hormones are readily absorbed through the skin, and applying creams is familiar and easily accomplished, assuring regular patient compliance.

2. Liver metabolism of hormone is minimized because red blood cells carry the hormone directly to its target organ passing the liver for at least one complete circulatory cycle, also known as the first pass effect.

3. Therapeutic levels are readily monitored by saliva testing.

Many over-the-counter progesterone creams are available, some excellent and well tolerated, while others lack quality control and contain preservatives and fragrances that can compromise absorption and lead to skin irritation. Fortunately, there are compounding pharmacists who can formulate a prescription for topically applied hormones. There is a surprisingly large contingent of pharmacists who tailor individual hormone prescriptions. You probably have one in your neighborhood (*see* www.iacprx.org for a referral). The listed compounding pharmacists use only USP (United States Pharmacopoeia) micronized progesterone and other pure hormones, making them the preferred source for bioidentical hormones. Most of these pharmacists will mail the prescription directly to your patient. It is to your advantage to find and work with local compounding pharmacists. They will often reciprocate with patient referrals. We routinely learn about important new information from our compounding pharmacists.

Sub-lingual

Sub-lingual application is popular with some practitioners, because it is also an effective hormone delivery method. However, because there is no effective method for monitoring therapeutic levels, this route of administration has limitations. Using this mode of administration leaves residual hormone in the saliva after dosing, causing false values on saliva tests. Another consideration is the unknown amount of the preparation unintentionally swallowed. The swallowed portion is essentially wasted or, as in the case of estradiol, can be detrimental because it lowers insulin-like growth factor one (IGF-1) a mediator of HGH.

Bioidentical Treatment Protocols

The following dosages, proven over the years to be effective, were taught to us by our mentors, including John Lee, MD, author of *Natural Progesterone: The Multiple Roles of a Remarkable Hormone* and other books on hormone balancing.

Progesterone

Perimenopausal woman interested in conception

USP Progesterone 20–30 mg in a transdermal base (e.g., Vanpen) applied beginning day 14 of the menstrual cycle, or the latter two weeks of menstrual cycle if longer or shorter than 28 days. Note: Do not stop the progesterone until menstruation begins or there is a negative pregnancy test. Once pregnancy is established continue topical progesterone at least until delivery. Rotate application daily to a thin region of the body: inner wrist, behind knees, upper inner arm, or upper chest. Dose may be given qd or split into bid application as preferred by provider and patient.

Example script: P4 25 mg/ml, #30, Sig: ½ ml bid or 1 ml qd (day 15 through 28). This should take the patient up to the two-month retest interval.

Perimenopausal woman NOT interested in conception

USP Progesterone 20–30 mg in a transdermal base (e.g., Vanpen) applied between periods, usually day 3 through 28 of the menstrual cycle. In other words, apply on days not menstruating. Rotate application daily to a thin region of the body: inner wrist, behind knees, upper inner arm, or upper chest.

Example script: P4 25 mg/ml, #30, Sig: ½ ml bid or 1 ml qd (day 3 through 28). You may want to give two refills, which will take the patient up to the two-month retest interval.

Postmenopausal woman

USP Progesterone 20–30 mg in a transdermal base (e.g., Vanpen) applied daily. Some providers prefer to cycle dosage, three weeks on and one week off, others recommend continuing daily doses. Rotate application daily to a thin region of the body: inner wrist, behind knees, upper inner arm, or upper chest.

Example scripts: P4 25 mg/ml, #30, Sig: ½ ml bid, qd, or alternatively, Sig: ½ ml bid or 1 ml qd (3 weeks on, 1 week off). You may want to give two refills, which will take the patient up to the two-month retest interval.

Bi-Estrogen (Bi-Est)

Perimenopausal woman interested in conception

USP Estriol (E3) and estradiol (E2) combination: 1 mg (E3:E2; 4:1) in a transdermal base (e.g., Vanpen) applied day 1 through 12 of the menstrual cycle. Rotate application daily to a thin region of the body: inner wrist, behind knees, upper inner arm, or upper chest. Dose may be given qd or split into bid application as preferred by provider and patient.

Example script: Bi-Est 1 mg (E3:E2; 4:1)/ml, #12, Sig: ½ ml bid or 1 ml qd (day 1 through 12). You may want to give two refills, which will take the patient up to the two-month retest interval.

Perimenopausal woman NOT interested in conception

USP Estriol (E3) and estradiol (E2) combination: 1 mg (E3:E2; 4:1) in a transdermal base (e.g., Vanpen) applied day 1 through 25 of the menstrual cycle. Rotate application daily to a thin region of the body: inner wrist, behind knees, upper inner arm, or upper chest. Dose may be given qd or split into bid application as preferred by provider and patient.

Example script: Bi-Est 1 mg (E3:E2; 4:1)/ml, #30, Sig: ½ ml bid or 1 ml qd (day 1 through 25). You may want to give two refills, which will take the patient up to the two-month retest interval.

Postmenopausal woman

USP Estriol (E3) and estradiol (E2) combination: 1 mg (E3:E2; 4:1) in a transdermal base (e.g., Vanpen) applied daily. Some providers prefer to cycle dosage, 3 weeks on and 1 week off, while others recommend continuous daily dosing. Rotate application daily to a thin region of the body: inner wrist, behind knees, upper inner arm, or upper chest.

Example scripts: Bi-Est 1 mg (E3:E2; 4:1)/ml, #30, Sig: ½ ml bid or 1 ml qd, or alternatively, Sig: ½ ml bid or 1 ml qd (3 weeks on, 1 week off). You may want to give two refills, which will take the patient up to the two-month retest interval.

Testosterone

USP testosterone: 0.5 to 1.5 mg in a transdermal base (e.g. Vanpen) applied daily. Some providers prefer to cycle dosage, 3 weeks on and 1 week off, while others recommend continuous daily dosing. Rotate application daily to a thin region of the body: inner wrist, behind knees, upper inner arm or upper chest.

Example scripts: Testosterone 0.5 mg/ml, #30, Sig: ½ ml bid or 1 ml qd; or alternatively, Sig: ½ ml bid or 1 ml qd (3 weeks on, 1 week off). You may want to give two refills, which will take the patient up to the two-month retest interval.

DHEA

USP DHEA: 5–10 mg in a transdermal base (e.g., Vanpen) applied daily. Rotate application daily to a thin region of the body: inner wrist, behind knees, upper inner arm, or upper chest.

Example scripts: DHEA 5 mg/ml, #30, Sig: ½ ml bid or 1 ml qd. You may want to give two refills, which will take the patient up to the two-month retest interval. Note: Due to conversion in the adrenal glands, DHEA supplementation will often raise testosterone levels, which eliminates the need for testosterone supplementation. DHEA supplementation may also raise estradiol levels and should be closely monitored.

Cortisol

Cortisol is available as Cortef or generic hydrocortisone (5 mg tablets) at any standard pharmacy. Compounding pharmacists can compound this into any concentration and include extended releasers to slow absorption. We have used both products with success. Also, there are supplement companies that provide animal adrenal extracts that contain unspecified amounts of cortisol (you can contact us for more details).

Our adrenal support dosing for someone in frank adrenal fatigue (flat line test) is: Cortisol 10 mg PO first thing in the morning with food and 5 mg PO at lunch, and rarely, 5 mg at 4 p.m. We rarely exceed 20 mg total daily dose, which is within physiologic range.[87] For an Addison's disease patient, of course, dosing will routinely exceed 20 mg, but rarely needs to exceed 50 mg per day.

Human Growth Hormone Deficiency (HGH)

Before supplementing with HGH, it is critical to first determine a patient's level of HGH production. The best test for determining this is a blood (serum) test. The level of insulin-like growth factor one (IGF-1), which is the biological mediator of HGH, is the preferred measurement for diagnosing and monitoring growth hormone deficiency. Unlike IGF-1, which fluctuates only 8% throughout a day, HGH fluctuates drastically throughout the day, making a single test result subject to error. Therefore, one would need several blood draws or a 24-hour urine test to establish the average production of HGH throughout the day (both methods are impractical and expensive.)

A single serum test is an effective approximation of overall HGH production. Once tested, the challenge is to optimize the HGH injection for the patient. Most laboratories report the IGF-1 reference ranges by age groups. This is well and good, but it only tells you that your patient is aging at the same rate as her peers. These ranges are often so broad that 99% of us fall within the range. To an uninformed provider, the reference range is often misconstrued as normal. For example, if the reference range for 60–70 year olds is 80 to 150 and your 62-year-old patient's IGF-1 level is 85 and falls within that range, you may tell the patient she is normal and not consider striving for a more youthful level that approximates that of a 40-year old, which is between 300 and 350. If this patient has a chronic disease, you may need to think outside of the box to help her achieve her goals.

Beware, there are many scams on the Internet regarding swallowing, snorting, or using transdermal HGH enhancers. Even some reputable pharmacists and physicians are recommending products other than injectable HGH. Though some of these products show benefits, the effects are transient, lasting only weeks or a few months. In the long run, these are a waste of money and expensive. Presently, subcutaneous injection is the only long-term option for effective HGH supplementation.

You may hear lengthy discussions regarding the best time for the injection: a.m. or p.m. In my personal experience, I started out dosing at bedtime, only to become disappointed with the IGF-1 response. Following encouragement from other experienced physicians, I switched to a.m. dosing and found significant increases with IGF-1 responses.

Dosing HGH should be individualized. Female dosing averages

2.4 iu/day (six days a week) and male dosing averages 1.2 iu/day. The dose is given by subcutaneous injection, in the belly around the navel works well.

A growth hormone secretague or sermorelin (injectable Geref) is an exciting product and is showing significant potential. Chemically, it is the first 29 amino acid segment in the sequence of growth hormone releasing hormone (GHRH) of the 44 amino acid sequence found in the body. This is the portion that stimulates the pituitary gland to produce and release growth hormone. The major advantage of sermorelin is the natural stimulation of growth production, which provides a more physiological level throughout the day as opposed to the square wave pattern associated with HGH injections.[88]

The proposed dosing ranges are 200–400 mcg/day SQ females, and 100–200 mcg/day SQ males. However, unlike HGH, it is best given at night and not skip a day. This may indeed be the next-generation product.

Combination Formulas

While all bioidentical hormones can be combined effectively into a single transdermal cream, it may be advantageous to prescribe the hormones individually in the first several months while finding the correct balance. Once combined into a single cream the absorption characteristics of each hormone may change slightly. DHEA is an exception because, in combination, it tends to compete with the other hormones for absorption, in particular, progesterone. We often limit the number of hormones in combination to three and give DHEA orally. Providers tend to be split evenly on which approach is best—as are we. You will have to find the approach that best suits you and your patients. We have found the following combination examples to effectively correct hormone imbalances for postmenopausal women:

Postmenopausal woman

Bi-Est 1 mg (E3:E2; 4:1)/ml, P4 25 mg, testosterone 0.5 mg/ml, #30, Sig: ½ ml bid or 1 ml qd or alternatively: Sig: ½ ml bid or 1 ml qd (3 wks on, 1 wk off). You may want to give two refills, which will take the patient up to the two-month retest interval. Note: DHEA, if needed, is best given separately and orally in order to eliminate absorption competition with progesterone.

Hormone Prescriptions and Their Percentages

Compounding pharmacist formulate creams by gram weight, which is often on the prescription label. You can write the script in mg/gm, mg/ml, or percentage depending upon your preference. The conversions below will help you understand the mg/gm or ml.

Conversion for All Hormone Creams	
Testosterone	1 mg/gm = 0.1% cream
	0.5 mg/gm = 0.05% cream
Note: A 0.05% cream is the recommended starting female dosage	
Bi-Est (4:1)	1 mg/gm = 0.1% cream
Progesterone	20 mg/gm = 2% cream

Side Effects

Because of their effectiveness, bioidentical supplementation needs to be monitored closely. If excess hormone is given, even in a bioidentical form, it can produce unwanted side effects. For example, if estrogen is given in excess of progesterone, the imbalance may lead to increase risk of breast cancer, as it would if the imbalance were occurring with a biological imbalance. Excess testosterone may lead to facial hair and scalp hair loss. Furthermore, excess hormone may cause a reduction in receptors on target organ membranes, which often causes a return of symptoms encouraging a dose increase, creating a vicious cycle. Another reason why patients should be tested prior to supplementation is to establish the exact nature and extent of the deficiencies. This assures a correct formulation and a safe and effective regimen. Baseline testing should always be followed with regular subsequent testing to monitor for the appropriate therapeutic levels. We recommend retesting every two months until balanced, and every 6–12 months thereafter.

In Summary

With the information in this book, you are ready to join the thousands of physicians who have discovered the satisfaction and success of treating patients with bioidentical hormones. Your practice will likely grow rapidly as word spreads that there is a physician in the community who will listen and work with patients interested in preventing disease and rebalancing their physiology to a more youthful state. You no longer need to prescribe harmful medications that do little more than cover up symptoms and lead to side effects that require yet another drug, and then another.

You will become a healer, which is most likely the reason you went to medical school in the first place. Dare to be the best physician you can; above all, do no harm. Though you may feel like the Lone Ranger as you make this transition, don't worry. You are not alone and your practice will reward you beyond words. We feel blessed to have the professional lives we live. Come join us!

Appendix A
Resources & Tools
Stacking the Deck

Hormone Testing Resources
To purchase Labrix Clinical Service's saliva hormone test kits, please contact Labrix at 1-877-656-9596 for retailers in your local area.

Compounding Pharmacies
1. The yellow pages can be very helpful. Look under Compounding Pharmacies. We try to support local compounding pharmacists whenever possible.
2. International Academy of Compounding Pharmacists is the best resource for a national search: www.iacprx.org

Locating a Practitioner Near You
1. American College for Advancement in Medicine: www.acam.org (A fellowship of complementary physicians—mainly MDs)
2. American Association of Naturopathic Physicians: www.naturopathic.org

Recommended Reading and Resources
Books

Barnes, Broda. *Hypothyroidism: The Unsuspected Illness*. New York, NY: HarperCollins. 1976.

Black, Jessica K. *The Anti-Inflammation Diet and Recipe Book*. Alameda, CA: Hunter House Publishers. 2006.

Brownstein, David. *Iodine: Why You Need It, Why You Can't Live Without It*. 2nd ed. West Bloomfield, MI: Medical Alternative Press. 2006.

Campbell CT, Thomas M, Campbell II, Robbins J; Lyman H. *The China Study: The Most Comprehensive Study of Nutrition Ever Conducted and the Startling Implications for Diet, Weight Loss and Long-term Health*. Dallas, TX: BenBella Books. 2006.

DesMaisons, Kathleen. *The Sugar Addict's Total Recovery Program*. New York, NY: Ballantine Books. 2002.

———. *Potatoes Not Prozac: A Natural Seven-Step Dietary Plan to Stabilize the Level of Sugar in Your Blood, Control Your Cravings and Lose Weight, and Recognize How Foods Affect the Way You Feel*. New York, NY: Simon Schuster. 1999.

Esselstyn, Caldwell B. *Prevent and Reverse Heart Disease*. New York, NY: Avery. 2007.

Jeffries, William Mck. *The Safe Uses of Cortisol*. 2nd ed. Springfield, IL: Charles C. Thomas. 1996.

Lee, John. *What Your Doctor May Not Tell You About Menopause: The Breakthrough Book on Natural Hormone Balance*. New York, NY: Warner Books. 2004.

Rubin, Jordan, Brasco, Jordan. *Restoring Your Digestive Health: How the Guts and Glory Program Can Transform Your Life*. New York, NY: Twin Streams. 2003.

Starr, Mark. *Hypothyroidism Type 2: The Epidemic*. Irvine, CA: New Voice Publications. 2005.

Willcox, Bradley, Willcox, Craig D, Suzuki, Makoto. *The Okinawa Program: How the World's Longest-Lived People Achieve Everlasting Health—And How You Can Too*. New York, NY: Clarkson Potter. 2001.

Wilson, James. *Adrenal Fatigue: The 21st Century Stress Syndrome*. Petaluma, CA: Smart Publications. 2001.

Web Sites
American College for the Advancement of Medicine
www.acam.org

International Academy of Compounding Pharmacists
www.iacprx.org

The American Association of Naturopathic Physicians
www.naturopathic.org

Dr. John Lee Institute
www.drjohnleeinstitute.com

Appendix B
References

Introduction

1. Life tables for WHO member states. *World Health Organiza-tion.* Available at www.who.int/whosis/database/life_tables/life_tables.cfm. Accessed October 10, 2007.

2. National vital statistics reports. *National Vital Statistics System, National Center for Health Statistics, Centers for Disease Control and Prevention, U.S. Department of Health and Human Services.* 2006;54(14). Revised 2007.

Chapter 1

3. Gumpert DE. Hormone battle: big pharma vs. small biz. *Business Week Online.* April 13, 2006:15.

4. Setting the record straight. *CompoundingFacts.* Available at http://www.compoundingfacts.org/info.cfm. Accessed October 11, 2007.

5. North American Menopause Society's ties to Wyeth Pharmaceuticals. *CompoundingFacts.* Available at www.compoundingfacts.org/info.cfm?News_ID=90. Accessed October 11, 2007.

6. Wilson RA. *At Any Age, You Can Be Feminine Forever.* New York, NY: Pocket Books. 1968.

7. Wilson R. No more menopause? *Newsweek.* January 13, 1964:53.

8. Rossouw JE et al. Risks and benefits of estrogen plus progestin in healthy postmenopausal women: principal results from the Women's Health Initiative randomized controlled trial. *JAMA.* 2002;288(3):321–333.

9. Current use of HRT linked to increased risk of ovarian cancer and death in 'The Million Women Study.' *Formulary.* 2007. Available at http://www.formularyjournal.com/formulary/Medication+S afety+and+Reliability/Current-use-of-HRT-linked-to-increased-risk-of-ova/ArticleStandard/Article/detail/457006. Accessed November 14, 2007.

10. Ravdin P et al. A sharp decrease in breast cancer incidence in the United States in 2003. *Proceedings from the 2006 annual San Antonio Breast Cancer Symposium.* Abstract 5. San Antonio, Texas. Oral presentation, December 14, 2006.

11. Paige LK. Premarin, politics, and the public health: an expose revealing how politics trumped science at the FDA. *Citizens Against Public Waste.* Available at www.cagw.org/site/PageServer?pagename=reports_premarin. Accessed October 11, 2007.

12. Kurtzman NA. JNC redux. Joint National Committee. *Am J Kidney Dis.* 1998;31(5):866–867.

13. Beral V. Breast cancer hormone-replacement therapy in the Million Women Study. *Lancet.* 2003;362(9382): 419–427. Erratum in: *Lancet.* 2003;362(9390):1160.

14. Wilson R. No more menopause? *Newsweek.* January 13, 1964:53.

15. Wilson RA, Wilson TA. The basic philosophy of estrogen maintenance. *J Am Geriatr Soc.* 1972;20(11):521–3.

16. Lee J. *What Your Doctor May Not Tell You About Menopause.* New York, NY: Warner Books Hachette Book Group. 1996. Rev. ed. 2004.

17. Ribot C, Tremollieres F. Hormone replacement therapy in postmenopausal women: all the treatments are not the same. *Gynecol Obstet Fertil.* 2007;35(5):388–97.

18. The history of pharmacy. Available at http://www.lindsaydrug.com/newhist.htm. Accessed November 14, 2007.

19. Wyeth statement on the citizen petition filed with the FDA related to bio-identical hormone replacement. *Life Sciences World.* Available at http://www.lifesciencesworld.com/news/view/7405. Accessed November 14, 2007.

Chapter 2

20. Chang KJ, Lee TT, Linares-Cruz G, Fournier S, de Lignieres B. Influences of percutaneous administration of estradiol and progesterone on human breast epithelial cell cycle in vivo. *Fertil Steril.* 1995;63(4):785–791.

21. Leonetti HB, Longo S, Anasti JN. Transdermal progesterone cream for vasomotor symptoms and postmenopausal bone loss. *Obstet Gynecol.* 1999;94(2):225–228.

22. Malleson J. Climacteric stress: its empirical management. *Br Med J.* 1956;2(5006):1422–1425.

23. Lee J. *What Your Doctor May Not Tell You About Menopause.* New York, NY: Warner Books Hachette Book Group. 1996. Rev. ed. 2004.

24. Strum JM. Effect of iodide-deficiency on the rat mammary gland. *Virchows Arch B Cell Pathol Incl Mol Pathol.* 1979;30(2):209–220.

25. Abraham GE. The Safe and effective implementation of orthoiodosupplementation in medical practice. *The Original Internist.* 2004;11:17–36. Available at http://optimox.com/pics/Iodine/IOD-05/IOD_05.html. Accessed November 25, 2007.

26. Abraham GE, Flechas JD, Hakala JC. Optimum levels of iodine for greatest mental and physical health. *The Original Internist.* 2002;9:5–20. Available at http://optimox.com/pics/Iodine/IOD-01/IOD_01.htm. Accessed November 25, 2007.

27. Abraham GE. The safe and effective implementation of orthoiodosupplementation in medical practice. *The Original Internist.* 2004;11:17–36. Available at http://optimox.com/pics/Iodine/IOD-05/IOD_05.html. Accessed November 25, 2007.

28. Ribas-Fito N et al. Breastfeeding, exposure to organochlorine compounds, and neurodevelopment in infants. *Pediatrics.* 2003;111(5 Pt 1):580–585.

29. Charlier C et al. Breast cancer and serum organochlorine residues. *Occup Environ Med.* 2003;60:348–351.

30. Charlier CJ et al. Polychlorinated biphenyls contamination in women with breast cancer. *Clin Chim Acta.* 2004;347:177–181.

31. Ribas-Fito N et al. Breastfeeding and concentrations of HCB and p,p'-DDE at the age of 1 year. *Environ Res.* 2005;98:8–13.

32. Wetherill YB, Fisher NL, Staubach A, Danielsen M, de Vere White RW, Knudsen KE. Xenoestrogen action in prostate cancer: pleiotropic effects dependent on androgen receptor status. *Cancer Res.* 2005;65(1):54–65.

33. Starek A. Estrogens and organochlorine xenoestrogens and breast cancer risk. *Int J Occup Med Environ Health.* 2003;16(2):113–124.

34. Nelson JA. Effects of dichlorodiphenyltricholroethane (DDT) and polychlorinated biphenyl (PCB) mixtures on 17β-[3H]es-tradiol binding to rat uterine receptor. *Biochem Pharmacol.* 1974;23(2):447–451.

35. Ribas-Fito N et al. Breastfeeding, exposure to organochlorine compounds, and neurodevelopment in infants. *Pediatrics.* 2003;111(5 Pt 1):580–585.

36. Charlier C et al. Breast cancer and serum organochlorine residues. *Occup Environ Med.* 2003;60:348–351.

37. Charlier CJ, Alvert AI, Zhang L, Dubois NG, Plomteux GJ. Polychlorinated biphenyls contamination in women with breast cancer. *Clin Chim Acta.* 2004;347:177–181.

38. Ribas-Fito N, Grimalt JO, Marco E, Sala M, Mazon C, Sunyer J. Breastfeeding and concentrations of HCB and p,p'-DDE at the age of 1 year. *Environ Res.* 2005;98:8–13.

39. Ribas-Fito N et al. Breastfeeding, exposure to organochlorine compounds, and neurodevelopment in infants. *Pediatrics.* 2003;111(5 Pt 1):580–585.

40. Ribas-Fito N, Grimalt JO, Marco E, Sala M, Mazon C, Sunyer J. Breastfeeding and concentrations of HCB and p,p'-DDE at the age of 1 year. *Environ Res.* 2005;98:8–13.

41. Starek A. Estrogens and organochlorine xenoestrogens and breast cancer risk. *Int J Occup Med Environ Health.* 2003;16(2):113–124.

42. Ribas-Fito N et al. Breastfeeding, exposure to organochlorine compounds, and neurodevelopment in infants. *Pediatrics.* 2003;111(5 Pt 1):580–585.

43. Ribas-Fito N, Grimalt JO, Marco E, Sala M, Mazon C, Sunyer J. Breastfeeding and concentrations of HCB and p,p'-DDE at the age of 1 year. *Environ Res.* 2005;98:8–13.

44. Ribas-Fito N et al. Breastfeeding, exposure to organochlorine compounds, and neurodevelopment in infants. *Pediatrics.* 2003;111(5 Pt 1):580–585.

45. Charlier C et al. Breast cancer and serum organochlorine residues. *Occup Environ Med.* 2003;60:348–351.

46. Charlier CJ, Alvert AI, Zhang L, Dubois NG, Plomteux GJ. Poly-chlorinated biphenyls contamination in women with breast can-cer. *Clin Chim Acta.* 2004;347:177–181.

47. Ribas-Fito N, Grimalt JO, Marco E, Sala M, Mazon C, Sunyer J. Breastfeeding and concentrations of HCB and p,p'-DDE at the age of 1 year. *Environ Res.* 2005;98:8–13.

48. Starek A. Estrogens and organochlorine xenoestrogens and breast cancer risk. *Int J Occup Med Environ Health.* 2003;16(2):113–124.

49. Wetherill YB, Fisher NL, Staubach A, Danielsen M, de Vere White RW, Knudsen KE. Xenoestrogen action in prostate cancer: pleiotropic effects dependent on androgen receptor status. *Cancer Res.* 2005;65(1):54–65.

50. Starek A. Estrogens and organochlorine xenoestrogens and breast cancer risk. *Int J Occup Med Environ Health.* 2003;16(2):113–124.

51. Charlier CJ, Alvert AI, Zhang L, Dubois NG, Plomteux GJ. Poly-chlorinated biphenyls contamination in women with breast can-cer. *Clin Chim Acta.* 2004;347:177–181.

52. Charlier C et al. Breast cancer and serum organochlorine residues. *Occup Environ Med.* 2003;60:348–351.

53. Campbell CT, Thomas M, Campbell II, Robbins J, Lyman H. *The China Study: The Most Comprehensive Study of Nutrition Ever Conducted and the Startling Implications for Diet, Weight Loss and Long-term Health.* Dallas, TX: BenBella Books. 2006.

Chapter 3

54. Overweight and obesity: U.S. obesity trends 1985–2006. *Department of Health and Human Services. Centers for Disease Control and Prevention.* Available at www.cdc.gov/nccdphp/dnpa/obesity/trend/maps/index.htm. Accessed October 15, 2007.

55. Shomon M. Major reversal at American Association of Clinical Endocrinologists regarding TSH levels and diagnosing hypothyroidism. *Thyroid-Info.* Available at http://www.thyroid-info.com/articles/aacereversal.htm. Accessed November 25, 2007.

56. Cancer stat fact sheets: Cancer of the breast. *National Cancer Institute: SEER (Surveillance Epidemiology and End Results).* Available at http://seer.cancer.gov/statfacts/html/breast.html. Accessed November 25, 2007.

57. Beral V et al. Breast cancer and hormone-replacement therapy in the Million Women Study. *Lancet.* 2003;362(9382):419–427.

58. Chen CL, Weiss NS, Newcomb P, Barlow W, White E. Hormone replacement therapy in relation to breast cancer. *JAMA.* 2002;287(6):734–741.

59. Rossouw, JE et al. Risks and benefits of estrogen plus progestin in healthy postmenopausal women: principal results from the Women's Health Initiative randomized controlled trial. *JAMA.* 2002;288(3):321–33.

60. Heart disease. *Department of Health and Human Services: Centers for Disease Control and Prevention.* Available at http://www.cdc.gov/heartdisease. Accessed November 25, 2007.

61. Rossouw JE et al. Risks and benefits of estrogen plus progestin in healthy postmenopausal women: principal results from the Women's Health Initiative randomized controlled trial. *JAMA*. 2002;288(3):321–333.

62. Lee Wen-Sen, Harder JA, Yoshizumi M, Lee ME, Haber E. Progesterone inhibits arterial smooth muscle cell proliferation. *Nat Med*. 1997;3(9):1005–1008.

63. Rosano GM et al. Natural progesterone, but not medroxyprogesterone acetate, enhances the beneficial effect of estrogen on exercise-induced myocardial ischemia in postmenopausal women. *J Am Coll Cardiol*. 2000;36(7):2154–2159.

64. Ramon Calle J. Response to type 2 diabetes: epidemiologic trends, evolving pathogenic concepts, and recent changes in therapeutic approach. *South Med J*. 2005;97(11):1079–1087.

65. Overweight prevalence. *Department of Health and Human Services: Center for Disease Control and Prevention*. Available at http://www.cdc.gov/nccdphp/dnpa/obesity/childhood/prevalence.htm. Accessed November 25, 2007.

66. Advocacy news & updates: America's bone health: the state of osteoporosis and low bone mass. *National Osteoporosis Foundation*. Available at http://www.nof.org/advocacy/prevalence. Accessed November 25, 2007.

67. Chihara K et al. Efficacy and safety of growth hormone (GH) in the treatment of adult Japanese patients with GH deficiency: a randomized, placebo-controlled study. *Growth Horm IGF Res*. 2006;16(2):132–142.

68. Vining RF, McGinley RA, Maksvytis JJ, Ho KY. Salivary cortisol: a better measure of adrenal cortical function than Serum Cortisol. *Ann Clin Biochem.* 1983;20(Pt 6):329–335.

69. Gozansky WS, Lynn JS, Laudenslager ML, Kohrt WM. Salivary cortisol determined by enzyme immunoassay is preferable to serum total cortisol for assessment of dynamic hypothalamic-pituitary-adrenal axis activity. *Clin Endocrinol.* 2005;63(3):336–341.

Chapter 4

70. O'Leary P, Feddema P, Chan K, Taranto M, Smith M, Evans S. Salivary, but not serum or urinary levels of progesterone are elevated after topical application of progesterone cream to pre- and post-menopausal women. *Clin Endocrinol (Oxf).* 2000;53(5):615–620.

71. Vining RF, McGinley RA, Maksvytis JJ, Ho KY. Salivary cortisol: a better measure of adrenal cortical function than serum. *Ann Clin Biochem.* 1983;20:329–335.

72. Gozansky WS, Lynn JS, Laudenslager ML, Kohrt WM. Salivary cortisol determined by enzyme immunoassay is preferable to serum total cortisol for assessment of dynamic hypothalamic-pituitary-adrenal axis activity. *Clin Endocrinol.* 2005;63:336–341.

Chapter 5

73. Willcox B, Willcox CD, Suzuki M. *The Okinawa Program: How the World's Longest-Lived People Achieve Everlasting Health— And How You Can Too.* New York, NY: Clarkson Potter. 2001.

74. Kow LM, Devidze N, Pataky S, Shibuya I, Pfaff DW. Acute estradiol application increases inward and decreases outward whole-

cell currents of neurons in rat hypothalamic ventromedial nucleus. *Brain Res.* 2006;1116(1):1–11.

75. Duckles SP, Krause DN. Cerebrovascular effects of oestrogen: multiplicity of action. *Clin Exp Pharmacol Physiol.* 2007; 34(8):801–808.

76. Lee J, Zava D, Hopkins V. *What Your Doctor May Not Tell You About Breast Cancer: How Hormone Balance Can Help Save Your Life.* New York, NY: Warner Books. 2002.

77. Campbell CT, Thomas M, Campbell II, Robbins J, Lyman H. *The China Study: The Most Comprehensive Study of Nutrition Ever Conducted and the Startling Implications for Diet, Weight Loss and Long-term Health.* Dallas, TX: BenBella Books. 2006.

78. Wilson, J. *Adrenal Fatigue: The 21st Century Stress Syndrome.* Petaluma, CA: Smart Publications. 2001.

79. Hashizume K. Administration of recombinant human growth hormone normalizes GH-IGF1 axis and improves malnutrition-related disorders in patients with anorexia nervosa. *Endocr J.* 2007;54(2):319–327.

Chapter 6

80. U.S. life expectancy below that of 41 other nations. *Medical News Today: Public Health News.* August 15, 2007. Available at http://www.medicalnewstoday.com/articles/79570.php. Accessed November 25, 2007.

81. U.S. infant death rate ranks highest compared to other industrial-

ized nations. *AHN Media Corp.* November 12, 2007. Available at http://www.allheadlinenews.com/articles/7009130745. Accessed November 25, 2007.

82. Starfield B. Is U.S. Health really the best in the world. *JAMA.* 2000;284(4):483–485.

83. Starfield B. Is U.S. Health really the best in the world. *JAMA.* 2000;284(4):483–485.

Chapter 7

84. Sicotte NL et al. Treatment of multiple sclerosis with the pregnancy hormone estriol. *Ann Neurol.* 2002;52(4):421–428.

85. Jefferies, WM. *Safe Uses of Cortisol.* 2nd ed. Springfield, IL: Charles C. Thomas. 1996.

86. Walker RF, Bercu BB. Contemporary therapies in longevity: society for applied research in aging. *Evid Based Int Med.* 2004;1(3):217–222(6).

87. Wilson RA, Wilson TA. The basic philosophy of estrogen maintenance. *J Am Geriatr Soc.* 1972;20(11):521–523.

88. Walker RF. Semorelin: a better approach to management of adult-onset growth hormone insufficiency? *International Society for Applied Research in Aging (SARA).* Available at http://www.semorelin.info/semorelin-editorial. Accessed January 19, 2008.

Appendix C
Selected Bibliography

Cortisol Levels and Breast Cancer

Bower JE, Ganz PA, Aziz N, Olmstead R, Irwin MR, Cole SW. Inflammatory responses to psychological stress in fatigued breast cancer survivors: relationship to glucocorticoids. *Brain Behav Immun.* 2007;21(3):251–258.

Carlson LE, Campbell TS, Garland SN, Grossman P. Associations among salivary cortisol, melatonin, catecholamines, sleep quality and stress in women with breast cancer and healthy controls. *J Behav Med.* 2007;30(1):45–58.

Carlson LE, Speca M, Faris, Patel KD. One year pre-post intervention follow-up of psychological, immune, endocrine and blood pressure outcomes of mindfulness-based stress reduction (MBSR) in breast and prostate cancer outpatients. *Brain Behav Immun.* 2007;21(8):1038–1049.

McVicar A, Greenwood CR, Fewell F, D'Arcy V, Chandrasekharan S, Alldridge LC. Evaluation of anxiety, salivary cortisol and melatonin secretion following reflexology treatment: a pilot study in healthy individuals. *Complement Ther Clin Pract.* 2007;13(3):137–145.

Soygur H et al. Interleukin-6 levels and HPA axis activation in breast cancer patients with major depressive disorder. *Prog Neuropsychopharmacol Biol Psychiatry.* 2007;31(6):1242–1247.

Spiegel D. Giese-Davis J, Taylor CB, Kraemer H. Stress sensitivity in metastatic breast cancer: analysis of hypothalamic-pituitary-adrenal axis function. *Psychoneuroendocrinology.* 2006;31(10):1231–1244.

Salivary Cortisol Testing

Aardal-Eriksson E, Karlberg BE, Holm AC. Salivary cortisol—an alternative to serum cortisol determinations in dynamic function tests. *Clin Chem Lab Med.* 1998;36(4):215–222.

Gozansky WS, Lynn JS, Laudenslager ML, Kohrt WM. Salivary cortisol determined by enzyme immunoassay is preferable to serum total cortisol for assessment of dynamic hypothalamic-pituitary-adrenal axis activity. *Clin Endocrin (Oxf).* 2005;63(3):336–341.

Meeran K, Hattersley A, Mould G, Bloom SR. Venipuncture causes rapid rise in plasma ACTH. *Br J Clin Pract.* 1993;47(5):246–247.

Morgan CA 3rd et al. Hormone profiles in humans experiencing military survival training. *Biol Psychiatry.* 2000;47(10):891–901.

Vining RF, McGinley RA, Maksvytis JJ, Ho KY. Salivary cortisol: a better measure of adrenal cortical function than serum. *Ann Clin Biochem.* 1983;20(Pt 6):329–335.

Xenobiotics and Xenoestrogens

Charlier CJ, Alvert AI, Zhang L, Dubois NG, Plomteux GJ. Polychlorinated biphenyls contamination in women with breast cancer. *Clin Chim Acta.* 2004;347(1–2):177–181.

Charlier C et al. Breast cancer and serum organochlorine residues. *Occup Environ Med.* 2003; 60(5):348–351.

Nelson JA. Effects of dichlorodiphenyltricholroethane (DDT) and polychlorinated biphenyl (PCB) mixtures on 17β-(3H) estradiol binding to rat uterine receptors. *Biochem Pharmacol.* 1974;23(2):447–451.

Ribas-Fito N et al. Breastfeeding, exposure to organochlorine compounds, and neurodevelopment in infants. *Pediatrics.* 2003;111(5 Pt 1):580–585.

Ribas-Fito N, Grimalt JO, Marco E, Sala M, Mazon C, Sunyer J. Breastfeeding and concentrations of HCB and p,p'-DDE at the age of 1 year. *Environ Res.* 2005;98(1):8–13.

Starek A. Estrogens and organochlorine xenoestrogens and breast cancer risk. *Int J Occup Med Environ Health.* 2003;16(2):113–124.

Wetherill YB, Fisher NL, Staubach A, Danielsen M, de Vere White RW, Knudsen KE. Xenoestrogen action in prostate cancer: pleiotropic effects dependent on androgen receptor status. *Cancer Res.* 2005;65(1):54–65.

Oral Estrogen Effect on IFG-1 Levels

Bellantoni MF, Harman SM, Cho DE, Blackman MR. Effects of progestin-opposed transdermal estrogen administration on growth hormone and insulin-like growth factor-1 in postmenopausal women of different ages. *J Clin Endocrinol Metab.* 1991;72(1):172–178.

Cano A, Castelo-Branco C, Tarin JJ. Effect of menopause and different combined estradiol-progestin regimens on basal and growth hormone-releasing hormone-stimulated serum growth hormone, insulin-like growth factor-1, insulin-like growth factor binding protein (IGFBP)-1, and IGFBP-3 levels. *Fertil Steril.* 1999;71(2): 261–267.

Caufriez A et al. Modulation of immunoreactive somatomedin-C levels by sex steroids. *Acta Endocrinol (Copenh).* 1986;112(2):284–289.

Cook DM, Ludlam WH, Cook MB. Route of estrogen administration helps determine growth hormone (GH) replacement dose in GH-deficient adults. *J Clin Endocrinol Metab.* 1999;84(11):3956–3960.

Fonseca E, Ochoa R, Galvan R, Hernandez M, Mercado M, Zarate A. Increased serum levels of growth hormone and insulin-like growth factor-1 associated with simultaneous decrease of circulating insulin in postmenopausal women receiving hormone replacement therapy. *Menopause.* 1999;6(1):56–60.

Friend KE, Hartman ML, Pezzoli SS, Clasey JL, Thorner MO. Both oral and transdermal estrogen increase growth hormone release in postmenopausal women—clinical research center study. *J Clin Endocrin and Metab.* 1996;81(6):2250–2256.

Ho KK, Weissberger AJ. Impact of short-term estrogen administration on growth hormone secretion and action: distinct route-dependent effects on connective and bone tissue metabolism. *J Bone Miner Res.* 1992;7(7):821–827.

Kam GY, Leung KC, Baxter RC, Ho KK. Estrogens exert route- and dose-dependent effects on insulin-like growth factor (IGF)-binding protein-3 and acid-labile subunit of the IGF ternary complex. *J Clin Endocrinol and Metab.* 2000;85(5):1918–1922.

Lueng KC, Johannsson G, Leong GM, Ho KK. Estrogen regulation of growth hormone action. *Endocr Rev.* 2004;25(5):693–721.

Weissberger AJ, Ho KK, Lazarus L. Contrasting effects of oral and transdermal routes of estrogen replacement therapy on 24-hour growth hormone (GH) secretion, insulin-like growth factor-I, and GH binding protein in postmenopausal women. *J Clin Endocrinol Metab.* 1991;72(2):374–381.

Progesterone

Carmody BJ, Arora S, Wakefield MC, Weber M, Fox CJ, Sidawy AN. Progesterone inhibits human infragenicular arterial smooth muscle cell proliferation induced by high glucose and insulin concentrations. *J Vasc Surg.* 2002;36(4):833–838.

Chang KJ, Lee TT, Linares-Crus G, Fournier S, de Lignieres B. Influences of percutaneous administration of estradiol and progesterone on human breast epithelial cell cycle in vivo. *Fertil Steril.* 1995;63(4):785–791.

Cuchacovich Miguel, Tchernitchin A, Gatica H, Wurgaft R, Valenzuela C, Cornejo E. Intraarticular progesterone: effects of a local treatment for rheumatoid arthritis. *J Rheumatol.* 1988;15(4):561–565.

Hermsmeyer RK et al. Prevention of coronary hyperreactivity in preatherogenic menopausal rhesus monkeys by transdermal progesterone. *Arterioscler Thromb Vasc Biol.* 2004;24(5):955–961.

Leonetti HB, Longo S, Anasti JN. Transdermal progesterone cream for vasomotor symptoms and postmenopausal bone loss. *Obstet Gynecol.* 1999;94(2):225–228.

Lee JR. Osteoporosis reversal: The role of progesterone. Published in the *International Clinical Nutrition Review*. 1990;10(3). Available at: http://www.naturodoc.com/library/hormones/osteo_rev.htm. Accessed January 8, 2008.

Malleson J. Climacteric stress: its empirical management. *Br Med J*. 1956;2(5006):1422–1425.

Mauvais-Jarvis P, Kuttenn F, Baudot N. Inhibition of testosterone conversion to dihydrotestosterone in men treated percutaneously by progesterone. *J Clin Endocrinol Metab*. 1974;38(1):142–147.

Rosano GM et al. Natural progesterone, but not medroxyprogesterone acetate, enhances the beneficial effect of estrogen on exercise-induced myocardial ischemia in postmenopausal women. *J Am Coll Cardiol*. 2000;36(7):2154–2159.

Sitruk-Ware et al. Treatment of benign breast disease by progesterone applied topically. In: *International Symposium on Percutaneous Absorption of Steroids*. Academic Press; 1980:219–229.

Stanczyk FZ, Paulson RJ, Roy S. Percutaneous administration of progesterone: blood levels and endometrial protection. *Menopause*. 2005;12(2):232–237.

Vining RF, McGinley RA. Hormones in saliva. *Crit Rev Clin Lab Sci*. 1986;23(2):95–146.

Wen-Sen L, Harder JA, Yoshizumi M, Lee ME, Haber E. Progesterone inhibits arterial smooth muscle cell proliferation. *Nat Med*. 3(9):1005–1008.

Wren BG, McFarland K, Edwards L. Micronized transdermal progesterone and endometrial response. *Lancet.* 1999;354(9188): 1447–1448.

Progesterone and Breast Cancer

Campagnoli C, Abba C, Ambroggio S, Peris C. Pregnancy, progesterone and progestins in relation to breast cancer risk. *J Steroid Biochem Mol Biol.* 2005;97(5):441–450.

Chang KJ, Lee TT, Linares-Cruz G, Fournier S, de Lignieres B. Influences of percutaneous administration of estradiol and progesterone on human breast epithelial cell cycle in vivo. *Fertil Steril.* 1995;63(4):785–791.

Cowan LD et al. Breast cancer incidence in women with a history of progesterone deficiency. *Am J Epidemiol.* 1981;114(2):209–217.

Desreux J et al. Progesterone receptor activation: An alternative to SERMs in breast cancer. *Eur J Cancer.* 2000;36(Suppl 4):S90–91.

Foidart JM et al. Estradiol and progesterone regulate the proliferation of human breast epithelial cells. *Fertil Steril.* 1998;69(5):963–969.

Formby B, Wiley TS. Bcl-2, survivin and variant CD44 v7-v10 are downregulated and p53 is upregulated in breast cancer cells by progesterone: Inhibition of cell growth and induction of apoptosis. *Mol Cell Biochem.* 1999;202(1–2):53–61.

Formby B, Wiley TS. Progesterone inhibits growth and induces apoptosis in breast cancer cells: Inverse effects on Bcl-2 and p53. *Ann Clin Lab Sci.* 1998;28(6):360–369.

Fournier A, Berrino F, Riboli E, Avenel V, Clavel-Chapelon F. Breast cancer risk in relation to different types of hormone replacement therapy in the E3N-EPIC cohort. *Int J Cancer.* 2005;114(3):448–454.

Horita K, Inase N, Miyake S, Formby B, Toyoda H, Yoshizawa Y. Progesterone induces apoptosis in malignant mesothelioma cells. *Anticancer Res.* 2001;21(6A):3871–3874.

Kaaks R et al. Serum sex steroids in premenopausal women and breast cancer risk within the European prospective investigation into cancer and nutrition (EPIC). *J Natl Cancer Inst.* 2005;97(10):755–765.

Laidlaw IJ, Clarke RB, Howell A, Owen AW, Potten CS, Anderson E. The proliferation of normal breast tissue implanted into athymic nude mice is stimulated by estrogen, but not progesterone. *Endocrinology.* 1995;136(1):164–171.

Lin VC et al. Progestins inhibit the growth of MDA-MB-231 cells transfected with progesterone receptor complementary DNA. *Clin Cancer Res.* 1999;5(2):395–403.

Malet C, Spritzer P, Guillaumin D, Kuttenn F. Progesterone effect on cell growth, ultrastructural aspect and estradiol receptors of normal human breast epithelial (HBE) cells in culture. *J Steroid Biochem Mol Biol.* 2002;73(3–4):171–181.

Mauvais-Jarvis P, Kuttenn F, Gompel A. Antiestrogen action of progesterone in breast tissue. *Horm Res.* 1987;28(2–4):212–218.

Missmer SA, Eliassen AH, Barbieri RL, Hankinson SE. Endogenous estrogen, androgen, and progesterone concentrations and breast cancer risk among postmenopausal women. *J Natl Cancer Inst.* 2004;96(24):1856–1865.

Mohr PE, Wang DY, Gregory WM, Richards MA, Fentiman IS. Serum progesterone and prognosis in operable breast cancer. *Br J Cancer.* 1996;73(12):1552–1555.

Nappi C, Affinito P, Di Carlo C, Esposito G, Montemagno U. Double-blind controlled trial of progesterone vaginal cream treatment for cyclical mastodynia in women with benign breast disease. *J Endocrinol Invest.* 1992;15(11):801–806.

Pasqualini JR, Paris J, Sitruk-Ware R, Chetrite G, Botella J. Progestins and breast cancer. *J Steroid Biochem Mol Biol.* 1998;65(1–6):225–235.

Plu-Bureau G, Le MG, Thalabard JC, Sitruk-Ware R, Mauvais-Jarvis P. Percutaneous progesterone use and risk of breast cancer: results from a French cohort study of premenopausal women with benign breast disease. *Cancer Detect Prev.* 1999;23(4):290–296.

Spicer DV, Ursin G, Pike MC. Progesterone concentrations—physiologic or pharmacologic? *Fertil Steril.* 1996;65(5):1077–1078.

Ticher A, Haus E, Ron IG, Sackett-Lundeen L, Ashkenazi IE. The pattern of hormonal circadian time structure (acrophase) as an assessor of breast cancer risk. *Int J Cancer.* 1996;65(5):591–593.

Progesterone and the Brain

Christenbury J. Progesterone shows promise as treatment for traumatic brain injuries. Emory University Health Sciences Center. EurekAlert. 2006. Available at: http://search.eurekalert.org/e3/query.html?qt=Progesterone+shows+promise+as+treatment+for+

traumatic+brain+injuries&col=ev3rel&qc=ev3rel&x=0&y=0.
Accessed January 8, 2008.

Jones NC, Constantin D, Prior MJ, Morris PG, Marsden CA, Murphy S. The neuroprotective effect of progesterone after traumatic brain injury in male mice is independent of both the inflammatory response and growth factor expression. *Eur J Neurosci*. 2005;21(6):1547–1554.

Stein DG. The case for progesterone. *Ann. N Y Acad. Sci*. 2005;1052: 152–169.

Stein DG. Progesterone exerts neuroprotective effects after brain injury. *Brain Res Rev*. 2007;Jul 27 [Epub ahead of print].

Stein DG, Wright DW, Kellermann AL. Does progesterone have neuroprotective properties? *Ann Emerg Med*. 2008;51(2):164–72.

Wright DW, Bauer ME, Hoffman SW, Stein DG. Serum progesterone levels correlate with decreased cerebral edema after traumatic brain injury in make rats. *J Neurotrauma*. 2000;18(9):901–909.

Progesterone and the Heart

Carmody BJ, Arora S, Wakefield MC, Weber M, Fox CJ, Sidawy AN. Progesterone inhibits human infragenicular arterial smooth muscle cell proliferation induced by high glucose and insulin concentrations. *J Vasc Surg*. 2002;36(4):833–838.

Hermsmeyer RK et al. Prevention of coronry hyperreactivity in preatherogenic menopausal rhesus monkeys by transdermal progesterone. *Arterioscler Thromb Vasc Biol*. 2004;24(5):955–961.

Lee Wen-Sen, Harder JA, Yoshizumi M, Lee ME, Haber E. Progesterone inhibits arterial smooth muscle cell proliferation. *Nat Med.* 1997;3(9):1005–1008.

Rosano GM et al. Natural progesterone, but not medroxyprogesterone acetate, enhances the beneficial effect of estrogen on exercise-induced myocardial ischemia in postmenopausal women. *J Am Coll Cardiol.* 2000;36(7):2154–2159.

Salivary vs. Serum Hormone Testing

Carey BJ, Carey AH, Patel S, Carter G, Studd JW. A study to evaluate serum and urinary hormone levels following short and long term administration of two regimens of progesterone cream in postmenopausal women. *BJOG.* 2000;107(6):722–726.

Chang KJ, Lee TT, Linares-Cruz G, Fournier S, de Lignieres B. Influences of percutaneous administration of estradiol and progesterone on human breast epithelial cell cycle in vivo. *Fertil Steril.* 1995;63(4):785–791.

Devenuto F, Ligon DF, Friedrichsen DH, Wilson HL. Human erythrocyte membrane uptake of progesterone and chemical alterations. *Biochim Biophys Acta.* 1969;193(1):36–47.

Gandara B, Leresche L, Mincl L. Patterns of salivary estradiol and progesterone across the menstrual cycle. *Ann N Y Acad Sci.* 2007;1098: 446–450.

Gann PH, Giovanazzi S, Van Horn L, Branning A, Chatterton RT Jr. Saliva as a medium for investigating intra- and interindividual differences in sex hormone levels in premenopausal women. *Cancer Epidemiol Biomarkers Prev.* 2001;10(1):59–64.

Gozansky WS, Lynn JS, Saudenslager ML, Kohrt WM. Salivary cortisol determined by enzyme immunoassay is preferable to serum total cortisol for assessment of dynamic hypothalamic-pituitary-adrenal axis activity. *Clin Endocrinol (Oxf)*. 2005;63(3):336–341.

Leonetti HB, Wilson KJ, Anasti JN. Topical progesterone cream has an antiproliferative effect on estrogen-stimulated endometrium. *Fertil Steril*. 2003;79(1):221–222.

Morley JE, Perry HM 3rd, Patrick P, Dollbaum CM, Kells JM. Validation of salivary testosterone as a screening test for male hypogonadism. *Aging Male*. 2006;9(3):165–169.

O'Leary P, Feddema P, Chan K, Taranto M, Smith M, Evans S. Salivary, but not serum or urinary levels of progesterone are elevated after topical application of progesterone one cream to pre- and postmenopausal women. *Clin Endocrinol (Oxf)*. 2005;53(5):615–620.

Stanczyk FZ, Paulson RJ, Roy S. Percutaneous administration of progesterone: blood levels and endometrial protection. *Menopause*. 2005;12(2):232–237.

Vining RF, McGinley RA. Hormones in saliva. *Crit Rev Clin Lab Sci*. 1986;23(2):95–146.

Vining RF, McGinley RA, Maksvytis JJ, Ho KY. Salivary cortisol: a better measure of adrenal cortical function than serum. *Ann Clin Biochem*. 1983;20(Pt 6):329–335.

Webley GE, Edwards R. Direct assay for progesterone in saliva: comparison with a direct serum assay. *Ann Clin Biochem*. 1985;22(Pt 6):579–585.

Wren BG, McFarland K, Edwards L. Micronised transdermal progesterone and endometrial response. *Lancet.* 1999;354(9188): 1447–1448.

Testosterone: Saliva vs. Serum Testing

Khan-Dawood FS, Choe JK, Dawood MY. Salivary and plasma bound and "free" testosterone in men and women. *Am J Obstet Gynecol.* 1984;148(4):441–445.

Morley JE, Perry HM 3rd, Patrick P, Dollbaum CM, Kells JM. Validation of salivary testosterone as a screening test for male hypogonadism. *Aging Male.* 2006;9(3):165–169.

Ohzeki T, Manella B, Gubelin-De Campo C, Zachmann M. Salivary testosterone concentrations in prepubertal and pubertal males: comparison with total and free plasma testosterone. *Horm Res.* 1991;36(5–6):235–237.

Pitteloud N et al. Increasing insulin resistance is associated with a decrease in Leydig cell testosterone secretion in men. *J Clin Endocrinol Metab.* 2005;90(5):2636–2641.

Sannikka E, Terho P, Suominen J, Santti R. Testosterone concentrations in human seminal plasma and saliva and its correlation with non-protein-bound and total testosterone levels in serum. *Int J Androl.* 1983;6(4):319–330.

Wang C, Plymate S, Nieschlag E, Paulsen CA. Salivary testosterone in men: Further evidence of a direct correlation with free serum testosterone. *J Clin Endocrinol Metab.* 1981;53(5):1021–1024.

Timing of Surgery for Breast Cancer

Badwe RA, Mittra I, Havaldar R. Timing of surgery with regard to the menstrual cycle in women with primary breast cancer. *Surgical Clin North Am.* 1999;79(5):1047–1059.

Fentiman, I. Timing of surgery and breast cancer. *Int J Clin Pract.* 2002;56(3):188–190.

Hrushesky, WJ. Menstrual cycle timing of breast cancer resection. *Recent Results Cancer Res.* 1996;140:27–40.

Kontos M, Fentiman IS. Perioperative endocrine status and prognosis in early breast cancer. *Breast J.* 2006;12(6):518–525.

Paradiso A, Serio G, Fanelli M, Mangia A, Cellamare G, Schittulli F. Predictability of monthly and yearly rhythms of breast cancer features. *Breast Cancer Res Treat.* 2001;67(1):41–49.

Wood PA, Hrushesky WJ. Sex cycle modulates cancer growth. *Breast Cancer Res Treat.* 2005;91:95–102.

Index